The QI/QM Troubleshooter

A STEP-BY-STEP GUIDE TO CMS' NEW REPORTING SYSTEM

Bonnie Foster, RN, BSN, MEd

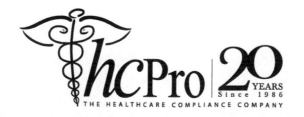

hcPro | 20 YEARS Since 1986
THE HEALTHCARE COMPLIANCE COMPANY

The QI/QM Troubleshooter: A Step-by-Step Guide to CMS' New Reporting System is published by HCPro, Inc.

ISBN 1-57839-782-0

Bonnie Foster, RN, BSN, MEd, Author
Janie Krechting, RNC, BSN, LNHA, MGS, Contributor
Elizabeth Petersen, Senior Managing Editor
Mike Mirabello, Senior Graphic Artist
Jean St. Pierre, Director of Operations
Patrick Campagnone, Cover Designer
Noelle Shough, Executive Editor
Paul Amos, Group Publisher

Arrangements can be made for quantity discounts. For more information, contact:

HCPro, Inc.
P.O. Box 1168
Marblehead, MA 01945
Telephone: 800/650-6787 or 781/639-1872
Fax: 781/639-2982
E-mail: *customerservice@hcpro.com*

Visit HCPro at its World Wide Web sites: *www.hcpro.com* and *www.hcmarketplace.com*

Contents

Contents

Introduction

Introduction

Definitions and terms used in this book

<u>ADJUSTED PERCENT:</u> Calculated by taking other health characteristics (covariates) and the national percent into account to adjust the observed percent:

> 5.2 Residents who have/had catheter inserted and left in bladder
>
> 8.1 Residents who have moderate to severe pain
>
> 9.3 Residents whose ability to move in and around room has worsened
>
> 13.1 Short-stay residents with delirium
>
> 13.3 Short-stay resident with pressure ulcers

<u>DATA QUALITY PROBLEMS:</u> Inconsistencies on the quality indicator/quality measure (QI/QM) reports that might indicate errors on the Minimum Data Set (MDS), i.e., denominator substantially exceeds or is substantially smaller than facility bed size, numerator exceeds resident population, or numerator for a certain QI/QM—restraints, for example—is "0," but there are residents wearing restraints.

<u>DENOMINATOR:</u> Number of facility residents who could have the QI/QM.

<u>GENERAL INDICATORS:</u> QI/QMs with some occurrence expected, i.e., prevalence of bowel or bladder incontinence or prevalence of pressure ulcers in high-risk residents.

<u>INCIDENCE:</u> Provides a description of what new conditions have occurred over the course of two assessments. (Residents who do not have target and prior assessments are excluded.) These may also have special exclusion criteria—i.e., 9.1 need for help with daily activities has increased, 9.4 e.g.,

decline in range of motion—both of these exclude residents whose previous assessment indicates no further decline is possible.

NUMERATOR: Number of residents who actually triggered a QI/QM.

OBSERVED PERCENT: Numerator divided by denominator multiplied by 100. This is the percent of residents who *could* have triggered and *did* trigger.

PERCENTILE: Facility's state rank, stated as a percent, on any given QI/QM. For example, if the facility's state percent is 75, then 75% of the other facilities in the state had a QI/QM score that was less than or equal to 75%.

PREVALENCE: QM/QI based on a single assessment. This provides the facility with percentages based on the target/current assessment.

RISK GROUPS: Residents in a low-risk group are less likely to trigger the QI/QM than those in a high-risk group. Risk groups are:

    2.2 Prevalence of behavior symptoms affecting others

    5.1 Low-risk residents who have lost control of bowels or bladder

    10.1 Prevalence of antipsychotic use in absence of psychotic diagnosis

    12.1 High-risk residents with pressure ulcers

    12.2 Low-risk residents with pressure ulcers

SENTINEL HEALTH EVENTS: QI/QMs that should occur very infrequently and will be investigated even if there is only one:

    5.4 Prevalence of fecal impaction

    7.3 Prevalence of dehydration

    12.2 Prevalence of pressure ulcers in low-risk patient

<u>THRESHOLDS:</u> Set points for each QI/QM that warrant further investigation. These are "flagged" on the Facility Quality Indicator/Measure Report as follows:

- Sentinel health events flagged if numerator is greater than "0"
- All other indicators/measures "flagged" if state percentile is greater than or equal to "90"

QI/QM: An overview

QI/QM: An overview

This manual is intended as a guide to the Quality Indicator/Measure Report (QI/QM) system. It describes how a facility can access reports from the database, how it can utilize these reports in providing quality resident care, and how the state survey team will use the reports in the survey process.

History

In 1984, the Institute of Medicine sponsored a study to review the quality of care in nursing homes. The results of that study indicated that the quality of care in nursing homes throughout the United States was substandard. In some cases, it was even clear that wrongful death had occurred. The Institute of Medicine wrote a report that addressed the findings and made recommendations for improvement.

This report was submitted to Congress in 1987. The result was the Omnibus Budget Reconciliation Act of 1987, now called OBRA '87, and the intent of the legislation was to improve the quality of care in nursing homes.

As a result of the recommendation to develop a standardized assessment instrument for all nursing home residents throughout the country, e.g., the Minimum Data Set (MDS) was developed.

The government gave the University of Wisconsin and the Center for Health Systems Research and Analysis the charge of using the MDS to develop a system to measure quality of care in nursing homes. Their task was to determine indicators that would measure quality and then validate those measures. The result was the Quality Indicator system.

The QIs

The original Quality Indicator (QI) reporting system was introduced to nursing homes by the Centers for Medicare & Medicaid Services (CMS) to provide facility-specific reports. There were 11 domains and 24 QIs, four of them broken down into high- and low-risk. The QIs were intended for use with the chronic and long-term care population.

Shortly thereafter, a project team comprising staff from Abt Associates, the Hebrew Center for the Aged, the Center for Gerontology and Health Care Research at Brown University, and the University of Michigan was delegated the task of validating the Quality Indicators that were already being used and using the MDS to measure quality items that would be understood by the public. The result of this study was the Quality Measures.

The QMs

In 2002, CMS formally released the QMs, which were used in the Nursing Home Compare public reporting system. The QM system included both chronic care and post-acute care measures. There were six chronic care quality measures and four post-acute care quality measures. Chronic or long-term care residents are those who stay longer than 14 days; short-term or post-acute care residents stay 14 days or fewer.

> The major difference in the Quality Indicators and the Quality Measures was the intended audience. The QMs were developed for the general public and nursing home care consumers, the QIs for use by regulators.

With the creation of the QMs, two different quality measurement systems now existed: the QI system, which was geared to measure quality within the nursing home, and the QM system, geared to measure quality of care for public reporting.

The QI/QMs

The new QI/QM reporting system replaces the old QI system, consolidating the two reports. This new system includes all of the QMs and any of the QIs that were not replaced by the QMs.

The QI/QM has five new items. Two of the items are chronic care items involving residents who have moderate to severe pain and residents whose ability to move in and around their room has gotten worse. The other three new items are post-acute items involving short-stay residents with delirium, short-stay residents who have moderate to severe pain, and short-stay residents with pressure ulcers.

FIGURE 1.1

The QMs

Chronic Care Measures

Accidents

- 1.1 Incidence of new fractures
- 1.2 Prevalence of falls

Behavior/Emotional Patterns

- 2.1 Residents who have become more depressed or anxious
- 2.2 Prevalence of behavior symptoms affecting others
- 2.3 Prevalence of symptoms of depression without antidepressant therapy
- 2.2-HI High-risk
- 2.2-LO Low-risk

Clinical Management

- 3.1 Use of nine or more different medications

Cognitive Patterns

- 4.1 Incidence of cognitive impairment

Elimination/Incontinence

- 5.1 Low-risk residents who have lost control of their bowels or bladder
- 5.2 Residents who have/had a catheter inserted and left in their bladder

FIGURE 1.1

The QMs (cont.)

- 5.3 Prevalence of occasional or frequent bladder or bowel incontinence without a toileting plan
- 5.4 Prevalence of fecal impaction

Infection Control

- 6.1 Residents with a urinary tract infection

Nutrition/Eating

- 7.1 Residents who lose too much weight
- 7.2 Prevalence of tube feeding
- 7.3 Prevalence of dehydration

Pain Management

- 8.1 Residents who have moderate to severe pain

Physical Functioning

- 9.1 Residents whose need for help with daily activities has increased
- 9.2 Residents who spend most of their time in bed or in a chair
- 9.3 Residents whose ability to move in and around their room got worse
- 9.4 Incidence of decline in range of motion (ROM)

Psychotropic Drug Use

- 10.1 Prevalence of antipsychotic use, in the absence of psychotic or related conditions
- 10.1-HI High-risk

FIGURE 1.1

The QMs (cont.)

Psychotropic Drug Use

- 10.1-LO Low-risk risk
- 10.2 Prevalence of antianxiety/hypnotic use
- 10.3 Prevalence of hypnotic use more than two times in last week

Quality of Life

- 11.1 Residents who were physically restrained
- 11.2 Prevalence of little or no activity

Skin Care

- 12.1 High-risk residents with pressure ulcers
- 12.2 Low-risk residents with pressure ulcers

Post-Acute Care (PAC) Measures

- 13.1 Short-stay residents with delirium
- 13.2 Short-stay residents who had moderate to severe pain
- 13.3 Short-stay residents with pressure ulcers

How QI/QM reports are generated

The MDS is the source document used to generate the QI/QM report. Each nursing home determines which staff member will complete each MDS item. For example, Section E, Mood, is typically completed by the facility social worker. Section O, Medications, is generally assigned to a nurse.

After each item is complete, the MDS coordinator signs the form, indicating that the document is complete. The information is then entered into a computer and submitted electronically in the state database. The state database is programmed to generate seven reports.

Factors impacting the QI/QMs include the following:

1. The types of MDS assessment being submitted. Assessments are submitted according to regulatory criteria. These include an admission MDS, a quarterly assessment, and an annual assessment. Significant change in status assessments are required when a resident meets the criteria for a significant change. You can locate criteria for a significant change in status in the *Resident Assessment Instrument User's Manual,* Chapter two. Admission assessments do not allow for comparison of items over multiple assessments.

2. Comparison items. These indicators compare an individual resident's condition over more than one assessment. For example, if a resident's activities of daily living (ADLs) declined from one assessment to another, this would trigger the QI/QM. If the resident's ADLs did not change, then the QI/QM would not trigger.

3. Risk items. High-risk items are responses that place a resident as being at high risk for developing a condition. For example, if a resident has impaired mobility, is comatose, or is suffering from malnutrition, this would place the resident at high risk for developing a pressure ulcer.

4. Exclusions. Exclusions are items that eliminate a resident from being included in a specific QI. Consider QI/QM 9.2: Residents who spend most of their time in a chair. Residents who

are coded as comatose in item B1 of the MDS are excluded from this QI/QM. Therefore, it becomes critical that the staff is trained in how to code specific MDS items, as each impacts the QI/QM report and ultimately the state survey.

Example

Below is a sample of how an item from the MDS can be coded and how it would translate into the QI/QMs. This item will flag the QI/QM: 1.2 Prevalence of falls. MDS Item(s): See the items checked below

Section J. Health Conditions					
4.	Accidents	*(Check all that apply)*		Hip fracture in last 180 days	c.
		Fell in past 30 days	a. ✓	Other fracture in last 180 days	d.
		Fell in past 31–180 days	b.	None of the above	e.

It is important to understand that some QI/QMs are outcome-related and others are process-oriented. **Outcome** is the end resident-centered result. **Process** reflects care delivery systems.

An outcome indicator would be QI/QM 2.1: Residents who have become more depressed or anxious. A process indicator is QI/QM 2.4: Prevalence of depression without antidepressant therapy. There are several process problems that could be contributing to lack of treatment. Lack of assessment, failure to notify the physician, or resident refusal may be reasons that a resident with depression is not treated.

Each staff member completing an item on the MDS should be aware of the impact the response will have on the survey process, the QI/QMs, and reimbursement. MDS training must go beyond filling in each item on the tool. It should incorporate the impact of the item for the QI/QM reports, the reimbursement system, and the survey process.

QI DOMAINS—BASED ON THE MDS 2.0

1. Accidents

2. Behavior/Emotional Patterns

3. Clinical Management

4. Cognitive Patterns

5. Elimination/Incontinence

6. Infection Control

7. Nutrition/Eating

8. Pain Management

9. Physical Functioning

10. Psychotropic Drug Use

11. Quality of Life

12. Skin Care

13. Post-Acute Care Measures

Descriptions of the QI/QM Measures

Descriptions of the QI/QM Measures

Chronic Care Measures

Following is a description of each Quality Indicator/Quality Measure (QI/QM) for the long-term or chronic care skilled nursing facility (SNF) population.

> **Note:** Prevalence QI/QMs come from the target MDS assessment, e.g., the most recent. Incidence QI/QMs come from the prior MDS assessment, including both the target assessment and the assessment preceding the target assessment.

1.1 Incidence of new fractures (MDS items J4c and J4d)

Numerator: Residents with new fractures checked on target MDS; item J4c is checked on target assessment, not on prior assessments or item J4d checked on target MDS, not on prior assessments

Denominator: All residents with the target MDS and prior MDS with no fractures on the prior assessments. The QI/QM is not risk adjusted.

Exclusions: Residents who did not trigger (resident not included in numerator) the item or who were missing MDS data on items J4c/J4d on either target assessment or prior assessment.

Questions to ask regarding residents who triggered this QI/QM:

- Was the resident admitted with fracture?
- If the resident is on Medicare, does documentation reflect skilled care?
- Is restorative nursing a part of the care plan?
- Are there strategies in place to prevent further injury?
- Is there a fall-risk assessment if the fracture was caused by a fall?
- Is there documentation of care of incision/cast, etc. (if applicable)?

1.2 Prevalence of falls (MDS item J4a)

Numerator: Falls within past 30 days (item J4a checked on target assessment)

Denominator: All residents with a valid target MDS assessment; note that this QI/QM is not risk adjusted

Exclusions: Residents satisfying either of the following conditions:

- Target assessment is an admission assessment
- Item J4a has missing data on target

Questions to ask regarding residents who triggered this QI/QM:

- Was a fall risk assessment done?

- Did the facility follow F324 guidelines (i.e., checking medications for side effects, checking shoes, checking environment)?

- Are measures in place for prevention of further falls/accidents?

- Does documentation include mention of falls, resulting nursing measures, notification of family/physician, and an incident/accident report?

A note on using physical restraints (F221): Restraints do not make residents safe and there must be a medical reason for their use. It is not the device that makes a restraint, but rather how the device is used and how it affects the resident. For instance, "chair alarms" do not prevent falls—they simply tell the staff that the resident is up. If staff constantly tells the resident to "sit back down," then the staff's behavior and the chair alarms can be interpreted as a restraint. The chair alarms are useful for residents who are independent and need a reminder to wait for staff to ambulate or go to the bathroom.

2.1 Residents who have become more depressed or anxious (MDS item E1)

Numerator: Mood scale score greater on target MDS than on prior assessment

Denominator: All residents with a valid target MDS and prior assessment; note that this QI/QM is not risk adjusted

Exclusions: Residents satisfying any of the following conditions:

- Mood scale score missing on target
- Mood scale score missing on prior assessment and symptoms present on target MDS
- Mood scale score at maximum (value 8) on prior assessment
- Resident is comatose or status unknown on target MDS

Mood Scale Score definitions

Count the number of the following conditions that occur on the target MDS:

- Verbal expression of distress
- Signs of crying/tearfulness
- Motor agitation
- Leaving food uneaten on target or last full assessment (item K4c: This item is considered only if target assessment is quarterly and state quarterly assessment does not include item K4c)
- Repetitive health complaints
- Repetitive/recurrent verbalizations
- Negative statements
- Mood symptoms not easily altered

Questions to ask regarding residents who triggered this QI/QM:

- Is social service involved in the resident's care?
- Have you conducted a psychological evaluation with specific approaches for the care plan?
- Are reasons for resident's mood documented?
- Is the resident's physician/pharmacist involved?

(2.2-HI: High-risk; 2.2-LO: Low-risk) Prevalence of behavior symptoms affecting others (MDS items E4b, E4c, and E4d)

Numerator: Residents with behavior affecting others on target assessment (verbally abusive or physically abusive or socially inappropriate/disruptive behavior)

Denominator: All residents with a valid target assessment

Exclusions: Residents satisfying any of the following conditions:

- Target assessment is an admission assessment (AA8a = 01)

- Measure did not trigger (resident not included in numerator) and data is missing in items E4bA, E4cA, or E4dA

- Resident does not qualify as high-risk or there is missing data in items B2a, B4, I1ff, or I1gg (i.e., the risk group is unknown)

In this measure, there are three separate items: one for all residents, one for high-risk residents, and one for low-risk residents. The only difference among these three is the denominator definition:

Denominator for overall: Includes residents with target assessment with only the first two exclusions applied

Denominator for high-risk: Includes residents with target assessment who are defined as high-risk, with all three exclusions applied

Denominator for low-risk: Includes residents with target assessment who are defined as low-risk, with all three exclusions applied

Questions to ask regarding residents who triggered this QI/QM:

- Is social services involved with the resident's care?

- Have you used psychological consultation with specific approaches for care plan? It is important that the clinician conducting the consultation hold an exit interview with the staff to ensure that there is enough information for the care plan so that the facility can keep the resident and other residents safe.

- Have other residents been kept safe?

- Is there a behavior management program on the care plan?

- Does documentation reflect that the care plan is followed?

- Is the resident involved in appropriate activities?

2.3 Prevalence of symptoms of depression without antidepressant therapy (MDS items O4c and E2)

Numerator: Residents with symptoms of depression, defined as sad mood and any two of the following on the target assessment:

- Distress
- Agitation or withdrawal
- Unpleasant mood in the morning, or awake one period of the day or less and not comatose
- Suicidal thoughts or recurrent thoughts of death
- Weight loss

Denominator: All residents with a valid target assessment

Exclusions: Residents satisfying either of the following conditions:

- Target assessment is an admission assessment

- The measure did not trigger (i.e., the resident was not included in numerator) and following two conditions are both satisfied: missing MDS data in B1, E1a, E1g, E1j, E1n, E1o, E1p, E2, E4eA, K3a, N1a, N1b, N1c, N1d, or O4c; and the measure could have been triggered if there had been no missing data

Questions to ask regarding residents who triggered this QI/QM:

- Are activity programs meeting resident's needs?
- Does the resident have a history of depression?
- Are care/treatments/recreation planned in the afternoon and not in the morning, if needed?
- Has the resident experienced weight loss? If so, is the dietary department involved?
- Has social service looked at the resident's customary routine?
- Have you examined what helped the resident's depression before he or she came to the facility?
- Have you included input from the resident's physician and the pharmacy?

3.1 Use of nine or more different medications (MDS item O1)

Numerator: Residents who received nine or more medications during the target assessment

Denominator: All residents with a valid target assessment

Exclusions: Residents satisfying either of the following conditions:

- The target assessment is the admission assessment
- O1 has missing data on the target assessment

Questions to ask regarding residents who triggered this QI/QM:

- Has a pharmacist reviewed medications according to OBRA/PPS regulations?
- Have there been any "holidays" for drugs?
- Has resident refused any ordered medications?
- Can the resident's needs be met with food rather than drugs (e.g., bananas instead of potassium supplements)?

4.1 Incidence of cognitive impairment (MDS items B4 and B2a)

Numerator: Residents who were cognitively impaired on the target assessment and not on the prior assessment

Denominator: All residents with a valid target assessment and prior assessment who were not cognitively impaired on the prior assessment

Exclusions: Residents satisfying either of the following conditions:

- The measure did not trigger (the resident was not included in the numerator)
- There is missing data in items B4 or B2a on the target or prior assessments

Questions to ask regarding residents who triggered this QI/QM:

- Does the MDS match nurses' documentation?
- Does physician documentation match the MDS?
- Are all staff using MDS definitions in their notes (e.g., instead of charting "alert but confused," document "resident has a 1 in short-term memory")?

5.1 Low-risk residents who have lost control of their bowels or bladder (MDS items H1a and H2a)

Numerator: Residents who were frequently incontinent or fully incontinent on target assessment (item H1a = 3 or item H1b = 3 or 4)

Denominator: All residents with a valid target assessment and not qualifying as high-risk

Exclusions:

- Residents who qualify as high-risk: severe cognitive impairment on the target assessment (item B4 = 3 AND item B2a = 1) OR totally dependent in self-performance mobility ADLs (item G1aA = 4 or 8 AND item G1bA = 4 or 8 AND G1eA = 4 or 8)

- Residents satisfying the following conditions are also excluded:

  1. Target assessment is an admission assessment

  2. QM did not trigger (resident not included in the QM numerator) AND the value of item H1a or H1b is missing on the target assessment

  3. The resident is comatose (item B1 = 1) or comatose status is unknown (B1 = missing) on the target assessment

  4. Resident has indwelling catheter (H3d = checked) or indwelling catheter status is unknown (H3d = missing) on the target assessment

  5. Resident has an ostomy (H3i = checked) or ostomy status is unknown (H3i = missing) on the target assessment

6. The resident does not qualify as high-risk and either of cognitive impairment items (B2a or B4) are missing on the target assessment

7. The resident does not qualify as high-risk and any of the mobility ADLs (G1aA, G1bA, and G1eA) are missing on the target assessment

Questions to ask regarding residents who triggered this QI/QM:

- Has the resident's reason for loss of control been assessed?
- Has the resident been assessed for toileting programs?
- Is there documentation of the resident's treatment refusal or lack of cooperation?

5.2 Residents who have/had a catheter inserted and left in their bladder (MDS item H3d)

Numerator: Residents with indwelling catheters on target assessment (item H3d checked)

Denominator: All residents with a valid target assessment

Exclusions: Residents satisfying either of the following conditions:

- Target assessment is an admission assessment
- H3d is missing on the target assessment

Risk adjustment (covariates):

1. Indicator of bowel incontinence on the prior assessment (covariate = 1 if H1a = 4; covariate = 2 if H1a = 0, 1, 2, or 3)

2. Indicator of pressure ulcers on the prior assessment (covariate = 1 if M2a = 3 or 4; covariate = 0 if M2a = 0, 1, or 2)

Questions to ask regarding residents who triggered this QI/QM:

- Does the resident have a physician-documented diagnosis justifying the indwelling catheter?
- Are systems in place to prevent urinary tract infection?
- Is the resident properly hydrated?
- Are all aspects of catheter and related care documented (i.e., size, color of urine, cleaning, etc.)?
- Are staff performing catheter treatments according to policy guidelines and infection control practices?

5.3 Prevalence of occasional or frequent bladder or bowel incontinence without a toileting plan (MDS items H1b and H1a)

Numerator: Residents with no scheduled toileting plan and no bladder retraining program (neither H3a nor H3b is checked) on the target assessment and either or both of the following conditions are met on the target:

1. Occasional or frequent bladder incontinence (H1b = 2 or 3)
2. Bowel incontinence (H1a = 2 or 3)

Denominator: Residents with frequent incontinence or occasional incontinence in either bladder (H1b = 2 or 3) or bowel (H1a = 2 or 3) on the target assessment

Exclusions: Residents satisfying either of the following conditions:

- Target assessment is an admission assessment
- The measure did not trigger (resident not included in numerator) and there is missing data in either H3a, H3b, H1a, or H1b

Questions to ask regarding residents who triggered this QI/QM:

- Has an assessment for a toileting program been completed?
- Is there documentation of resident refusal or noncompliance in the medical record?
- Has the resident complained of staff not answering requests for the bathroom in a timely manner?
- Is there a policy and procedure for both bladder retraining and toileting in the facility?

5.4 Prevalence of fecal impaction (MDS items H2d) (sentinel health event)

Numerator: Residents with fecal impaction (H2d is checked) on the most recent assessment

Denominator: All residents with a valid target assessment

Exclusions: Residents satisfying either of the following conditions:

- Target assessment is an admission assessment
- H2d is missing on target assessment

Questions to ask regarding residents who triggered this QI/QM:

- Has the resident's physician been educated about sentinel events?
- Have residents with a history of fecal impaction been assessed?
- Does the care plan feature measures to prevent fecal impaction?
- Is there a standing order for constipation, laxatives, enemas, etc.?
- How do staff document bowel movements (i.e., on the CNA flowsheets)?
- Does nursing check the bowel record each shift every day?
- Has the facility asked the resident and family what they did at home to prevent fecal impaction and followed that routine?

6.1 Residents with a urinary tract infection (MDS item I2j)

Numerator: Residents with a urinary tract infection on the target assessment (item I2j checked)

Denominator: All residents with a valid target assessment

Exclusions: Residents satisfying either of the following conditions:

- The target assessment is an admission assessment
- I2j is missing on the target assessment

Questions to ask regarding residents who triggered this QI/QM:

- Is facility using the urinary tract infection definition from the *Resident Assessment Instrument (RAI) User's Manual*?
- Has the physician ordered lab tests?
- Is the urinary tract infection recurrent?
- Is there dietary involvement to ensure proper hydration?
- Has staff been trained in proper incontinence care and monitored/evaluated?
- Have residents who qualify been placed on toileting programs?
- Is there appropriate documentation in the medical record to reflect the above items?

7.1 Residents who lose too much weight (MDS items K3a)

Numerator: Residents who have experienced weight loss of 5% or more in the past 30 days or 10% or more in the past six months

Denominator: All residents with a valid target assessment

Exclusions: Residents satisfying any of the following conditions:

- The target assessment is an admission assessment.

- K3a is missing on the target assessment.

- Resident is receiving hospice care (item P1ao is checked) or hospice status is missing (item P1ao information is missing) on the target assessment or most recent full assessment. The P1ao value from the last full assessment is considered only if the target assessment is a quarterly assessment and the state quarterly assessment does not include P1ao.

Questions to ask regarding residents who triggered this QI/QM:

- Are residents being weighed according to recognized nursing standards?

- Is the resident's usual body weight and not his or her ideal body weight used?

- Is there proper documentation for explained weight loss (i.e., amputation, reducing diet, diuretic)?

- Was the resident assessed for conditions that put him or her at risk for weight loss (i.e., cancer, renal disease, Alzheimer's, infection, dehydration, swallowing problems, ill-fitting/missing dentures, abnormal lab values, mouth pain)?

- Is there medical director/physician/nursing involvement and is it on the care plan?

- Is special attention paid to residents who also flag dehydration, pressure ulcers, tube feeding, urinary tract infections, and pain?

- Is facility using nutritional supplements instead of encouraging residents to eat nutritionally sound meals?

- Are assistance/adaptive devices/proper positioning provided for residents during mealtime?

- Does medication interfere with eating (i.e., bad tasting, given right before meals so resident is too full to eat, etc.)?

- Does the care plan reflect proper interventions such as assistance needed, adaptive devices, and liberalized diet? Is the care plan followed by staff?

- Are there comfortable sound levels, adequate lighting, absence of odors, tables adjusted to accommodate wheelchairs, appropriate hygiene prior to meals, eyeglasses/dentures/hearing aids in place?

- Has anyone met with the resident council to see if there are any food/meal complaints?

- Are staff assigned to dining rooms for all meals seven days a week?

- How is staff monitoring the amount eaten? Is a point system used? If the resident has lost weight and the monitoring shows that the resident has eaten all food at all meals, ask the following: While there may be no food on the plate, how much food is on the resident's clothes/the floor/eaten by another resident? In addition, some residents request only a bowl of soup and sandwich for supper. Even if they eat all of this meal, it is still does not provide all their nutritional needs.

- Are plates being returned to the kitchen with 75% or more food uneaten? If the residents are not eating a certain food, check to see if it needs to be taken off the menu.

7.2 Prevalence of tube feeding (MDs items K5b)

Numerator: Residents with tube feeding (item K5b is checked) on target assessment

Denominator: All residents with a valid target assessment

Exclusions: Residents satisfying either of the following conditions:

- The target assessment is an admission assessment
- Item K5b is missing on target assessment

Questions to ask regarding residents who triggered this QI/QM:

- Does your facility have a policy and procedure for tube feeding?
- Do physician's orders state type of feeding, flushing, residual directions, etc.?
- Do nursing staff follow standards of practice (e.g., head of bed elevated, etc.)?
- Is the nursing staff monitored on a routine basis to ensure compliance with feeding?
- Has speech pathology been involved to see if the resident is able to eat by mouth?
- Do the resident and family members understand the importance of following guidelines (e.g., not giving anything by mouth if the resident is at risk for aspiration)?

7.3 Prevalence of dehydration (MDS items J1c and I3a–I3e) (sentinel health event)

Numerator: Residents with dehydration (output exceeds input) on the target assessment (item J1c is checked) or I3a–I3e = ICD-9 276.5 code

Denominator: All residents with a valid target assessment

Exclusions: Residents satisfying either of the following conditions:

- The target assessment is an admission assessment
- J1c is missing on target assessment

Questions to ask regarding residents who triggered this QI/QM:

- Is your facility using the *RAI User's Manual* definition for dehydration?

- If the resident was admitted with dehydration, is he or she being assessed to see if it has been resolved?

- Is there a policy for hydration in facility?

- Does the care plan reflect that residents are given fluids and not just offered fluids if they are cognitively impaired?

- Is special attention paid to residents who also have fecal impaction, weight loss, tube feeding, urinary tract infections, and pressure ulcers and residents who need help with daily activities?

- Does your facility use a baseline measurement for daily fluid needs?

- Does the care plan reflect existing clinical conditions and risk factors?

- Are the fluids given (i.e., caffeine) contributing to dehydration?

- If resident is on thickened liquids, are they being provided correctly?

- Is the room temperature contributing to dehydration?

- Can cognitive residents reach fluids and is there a policy of when water/ice is served?

8.1 Residents who have moderate to severe pain (MDS items J2a and J2b)

Numerator: Residents with moderate pain at least daily (item J2a = 2 and J2b = 2) OR horrible/excruciating pain at any frequency (item J2b = 3) on the target assessment

Denominator: All residents with a valid target assessment

Exclusions: Residents satisfying any of the following conditions:

- Target assessment is an admission assessment
- Either item J2a or item J2b is missing on the target assessment
- The values of items J2a and J2b are inconsistent (i.e., J2a = 0 and J2b is not blank or J2a > 0 and J2b = blank)

Risk adjustment (covariate): Indicator of independence or modified independence in daily decision-making on prior assessment:

- Covariate = 1 if item B4 = 0 or 1
- Covariate = 0 if B4 = 2 or 3

Questions to ask regarding residents who triggered this QI/QM:

- Does your facility have pain assessment forms for cognitive and non-cognitive residents?
- Is there a pain management program in place at the facility?
- Is pain medication given prior to therapy, meals, dressing changes, etc.?
- Is there documentation of pain medication/pain relief and is it on the care plan?
- Have alternate methods for pain relief, besides medication, been tried based on resident's customary routine?

9.1 Residents whose need for help with daily activities has increased (MDS items G1aA, G1bA, G1hA, and G1iA)

Numerator: Residents with worsening late-loss ADL self-performance scores at the target assessment relative to the prior assessment. Late-loss ADL dependence is considered increasing when there is a specified increase in dependence from the prior assessment to the target assessment, except when residents have reached their maximum late-loss. The QI/QM is triggered when AT LEAST TWO of bed mobility, transferring, eating or toileting increase one point or more, or AT LEAST ONE item increases two points or more.

Denominator: All residents with a valid target assessment and prior assessment

Exclusions: Residents meeting any of the following conditions:

- None of the four late-loss ADLs (items G1aA, G1bA, G1ha, and G1iA) can show decline because they already have a value of "4" or "8" on the prior assessment.

- The QM did not trigger (resident not included in numerator) AND there is missing data on any of the four late-loss ADLs on the target assessment or prior assessment.

- The resident is comatose (item B1 = 1) or comatose status is unknown (value for item B1 is missing) on the target assessment.

- The resident has end-stage renal disease (item J5c is checked) or end-stage renal disease is unknown (value for item J5c is missing) on the target assessment.

- The resident is receiving hospice care (item P1ao is checked) or hospice status is unknown (value for item P1ao is missing). The P1ao value from the last full assessment is considered only if the target assessment is a quarterly assessment and the state quarterly assessment does not include P1ao.

Questions to ask regarding residents who triggered this QI/QM:

- Has the resident been assessed for decline?
- Is the resident on a restorative program?
- Has the resident been seen by therapy, if indicated?
- Is there documentation of refusal of treatment/noncompliance in medical record?

9.2 Residents who spend most of their time in bed or in a chair (MDS item G6a)

Numerator: Residents who are bedfast (item G6a is checked) on the target assessment

Denominator: All residents with a valid target assessment

Exclusions: Residents meeting any of the following conditions:

- The target assessment is an admission assessment
- G6a is missing on the target assessment
- The resident is comatose (item B1 = 1) or comatose status is unknown (item B1 value is missing) on the target assessment

Questions to ask regarding residents who triggered this QI/QM:

- Are you using *RAI User's Manual* definitions?
- Does documentation provide reasons for resident's bed-bound status?
- Have there been any negative outcomes from this behavior? If so, are these outcomes documented?

9.3 Residents whose ability to move in and around their room got worse (MDS item G1eA)

Numerator: Residents whose locomotion self-performance is worse on the target assessment than on the prior assessment

Denominator: All residents with a valid target assessment and prior assessment

Exclusions: Residents satisfying any of the following conditions:

- The G1eA value is missing on the target assessment.

- The G1eA value is missing on the prior assessment and the G1eA value shows some dependence on the target assessment.

- The G1eA value on the prior assessment is "4" (total dependence) or "8" (activity did not occur).

- The resident is comatose (item B1 = 1) or comatose status is unknown (item B1 value is missing) on the target assessment.

- The resident has end-stage renal disease (item J5c is checked) or end-stage renal disease is unknown (value for item J5c is missing) on the target assessment.

- The resident is receiving hospice care (item P1ao is checked) or hospice status is unknown (value for item P1ao is missing). The P1ao value from the last full assessment is considered only if the target assessment is a quarterly assessment and the state quarterly assessment does not include P1ao.

Risk adjustment/covariates:

1. Indicator of recent falls on the prior assessment:

   - Covariate = 1 if items J4a or J4b are checked
   - Covariate = 0 if both items J4a and J4b are not checked

2. Indicator of extensive support or more dependence in eating on the prior assessment:

   - Covariate = 1 if item G1hA = 3, 4, or 8
   - Covariate = 0 if item G1hA = 0, 1, or 2

3. Indicator of extensive support or more dependence in toileting on the prior assessment:

   - Covariate = 1 if item G1iA = 3, 4, or 8
   - Covariate = 0 if item G1iA = 0, 1, or 2

Questions to ask regarding residents who triggered this QI/QM:

   - Was resident discharged from therapy and is now declining?
   - Is resident in a restorative program?
   - Has a physician documented a reason for the decline?
   - Has the resident been assessed for depression and pain?
   - Has there been an event that might explain this behavior (i.e., loss of a family member, etc.)?

9.4 Incidence of decline in range of motion (ROM) (MDS Items G4aA, G4bA, G4cA, G4dA, G4eA, and G4fA)

Numerator: Residents with increases in functional limitation in ROM between prior and target assessments. *Functional limitation in ROM defined as: If limitations in the neck, arm, hand, leg, foot, and others are summed on the prior and target assessments and sum increases, this QI/QM is triggered.*

Denominator: All residents with a valid target and prior assessments

Exclusions: Residents satisfying either of the following conditions:

- Resident with maximal loss of ROM on prior assessment
- Residents with missing data in items G4aA, G4bA, G4cA, G4dA, G4eA, or G4fA on target or prior assessments

Questions to ask regarding residents who triggered this QI/QM:

- Is resident receiving ROM care through nursing, restorative services, activities, etc.?
- Is there documentation of refusal or treatment/noncompliance by the resident?

10.1 Prevalence of antipsychotic use, in the absence of psychotic or related conditions (MDS items O4a)

Numerator: Residents receiving antipsychotics (item O4a $\geq$ 1) on target assessment

Denominator: All residents on target, except those with psychotic or related conditions

Exclusions: Residents satisfying any of the following conditions:

- The target assessment is an admission assessment

- Residents with one or more of the following on target or most recent full assessment:

    1. Items I3a–I3e ICD-9 codes are 295.**, -295.**, 297.**, or -298**
    2. Item I1gg: schizophrenia is checked
    3. Tourette's (items I3a–I3e ICD-9 = 307.23)
    4. Huntington's (items I3a–I3e ICD-9 = 333.4 or 333.40)

- Residents with hallucinations (item J1i is checked) on the target assessment

- Residents who do not trigger the measure (not included in numerator) and who have missing data in items O4a, I1gg, or J1i

- Residents who are not high-risk and following two conditions are satisfied: missing data on any of B2a, B4, E4bA, E4cA, E4dA and high-risk could have resulted if there had been no missing data

Risk adjustment: Based on denominator definition:

- High-risk: All residents, excluding those with psychotic/related conditions, with cognitive impairment and behavior symptoms affecting others with all five exclusions applied

 The QI/QM Troubleshooter

- Low-risk: All residents, excluding those with psychotic/related conditions, who do not qualify as high-risk with all five exclusions applied

Questions to ask regarding residents who triggered this QI/QM:

- Is your facility following guidelines for antipsychotic use outlined in the *State Operations Manual*?
- Is there pharmacy involvement?
- Is resident involved in restorative/activities/behavior management program, etc.?
- Is there documentation of the resident's behavior, cognition, etc.?

10.2 Prevalence of antianxiety/hypnotic use (MDS items O4b and O4d)

Numerator: Residents who received antianxiety medication or hypnotics (items O4b or O4d ≥ 1) on the target assessment

Denominator: All residents on the target assessment, except those with psychotic/related conditions

Exclusions: Residents satisfying any of the following conditions:

- The target assessment is an admission assessment

- Residents with one or more of the following on target or most recent full assessment:

  1. Items I3a–I3e ICD-9 codes are 295.**, -295.**, 297.**, or -298**
  2. Item I1gg: schizophrenia is checked
  3. Tourette's (items I3a–I3e ICD-9 = 307.23)
  4. Huntington's (items I3a–I3e ICD-9 = 333.4 or 333.40)

- Residents with hallucinations (item J1i is checked) on the target assessment

- Residents who do not trigger the measure (not included in numerator) and who have missing data in items O4b, O4d, I1gg, or J1i

Questions to ask regarding residents who triggered this QI/QM:

- Is the reason for medication use documented by physician and nurses?
- Have alternatives to medications been tried, with the successes/failures documented and included on the care plan?

10.3 Prevalence of hypnotic use more than two times in last week (MDS item O4d)

Numerator: Residents who received hypnotics more than two times in past week (item O4d > 2)

Denominator: All residents with a valid target assessment

Exclusions: Residents satisfying either of the following conditions:

- The target assessment is admission assessment
- Data for item O4d is missing on the target assessment

Questions to ask regarding residents who triggered this QI/QM:

- Have other measures been tried based on resident's customary routine (i.e., soothing baths, back rubs, etc.)?

- Is there documentation of the need for hypnotic medication with the successes/failures documented and included on the care plan?

11.1 Residents who were physically restrained (MDS items P4c, P4d, and P4e)

Numerator: Residents who were physically restrained daily on the target assessment (items P4c, P4d, or P4e = 2) Restraints are defined as items on the resident's trunk or limbs or device on a chair that prevents rising.

Denominator: All residents with a valid target assessment

Exclusions: Residents satisfying either of the following conditions:

- Target assessment is admission assessment
- QM did not trigger (resident is not included in QM numerator) AND value of P4c, P4d, or P4e is missing on the target assessment

Questions to ask regarding residents who triggered this QI/QM:

- Is the facility following the guidance set forth in F 221 of the *State Operations Manual?*

- Is there an assessment for at-risk residents and permissions/statements of risks given by resident/responsible party, if warranted?

- Have alternatives to restraints been tried?

- Is there documentation of restraint use and reduction and continued assessment in the medical record?

- Does the staff understand that it is not the device itself that constitutes a restraint, but rather what the device does to the resident?

- Does the facility understand the difference between marking side rails on the MDS under G6b as transfer, mobility devices and under P4 as restraints?

11.2 Prevalence of little or no activity (MDS item N2)

Numerator: Residents with little or no activity (item N2 = 2 or 3) on the target assessment

Denominator: All residents with a valid target assessment

Exclusions: Residents satisfying any of the following conditions:

- The target assessment is an admission assessment
- The resident is comatose (item B1 = 1) or data for items N2 or B1 is missing on the target assessment

Questions to ask regarding residents who triggered this QI/QM:

- Was resident's activity preference assessed?
- Does the activity routine follow resident's customary routine (i.e., staying in room reading if that was the past routine, etc.)?
- Is an activity calendar provided so the resident can make choices?
- Has the activity calendar been discussed at resident council meetings?
- Are there activities in the evening and on weekends?
- Are there appropriate activities for residents with dementia?
- Does the care plan reflect specific preferences?
- Are activities age/gender-specific?

12.1 High-risk residents with pressure ulcers (MDS items M2a and I3)

Numerator: Residents with Stage 1–4 pressure ulcers (item M2a > 0 or items I3a–I3e = ICD-9 707.0*) on the target assessment who are defined as high-risk. High-risk is defined as impaired in bed mobility or transfer; comatose; or suffering malnutrition on the target assessment

Denominator: All residents with a valid target assessment and any one of the high-risk criteria:

- Impaired in bed mobility or transfer on the target assessment (item G1aA = 3, 4, or 8 OR item G1bA = 3, 4, or 8)

- Comatose on the target assessment (item B1 = 1)

- Suffering malnutrition on the target assessment as indicated by I3a–I3e = ICD-9 260, 261, 262, 263.0, 263.1, 263.2, 263.8, or 263.9

Exclusions: Residents satisfying either of the following conditions:

- Target assessment is an admission assessment
- The QM did not trigger (resident not included in QM numerator) AND the value of item M2a is missing on the target assessment

Questions to ask regarding residents who triggered this QI/QM:

- Is your facility following the guidance set forth in F314 in the *State Operations Manual*?

- Do definitions provided match those on the MDS and in documentation?

- Is facility using an "at risk" form for assessment?

- Is there documentation of staff training on skin care, pressure points, tissue tolerance, nutrition guidelines, etc.?

- Are there prevention procedure guidelines in the facility policy manual? If so, are they followed and addressed in the care plan?

- Are interventions specific for the resident (such as resident's choices and advance directives) included in the care plan?

- Are pressure ulcers monitored by the physician?

- Are the specific guidelines for documentation set forth in F314 followed by the physician and by nursing staff?

- Are possible infections monitored and pain management measures employed?

- Is the facility familiar with possible other F-tags related to pressure ulcers (such as F501)?

- Is special attention paid to residents suffering from dehydration, fecal impaction, urinary tract infections, and weight loss, those with tube feeding, and those whose ADL assistance needs have increased?

- If the resident frequently sits in a chair, is the facility using other measures besides "microshifting" to relieve pressure?

- If the resident refuses prevention measures or treatment, is this documented in the clinical record?

12.2 Low-risk residents with pressure ulcers (MDS items M2a and I3) (sentinel health event)

Numerator: Residents with Stage 1–4 pressure ulcers (item M2a > 0 OR I3a–I3e = ICD-9 707.0*) on the target assessment who are defined as low-risk

Denominator: All residents with a valid target assessment defined as low-risk; low-risk residents are those who did not qualify as high-risk as defined in measure 12.1

Exclusions: Residents satisfying any of the following conditions are excluded from both risk groups (high and low):

- The target assessment is admission assessment

- The QM did not trigger (resident not included in QM numerator) AND the value of item M2a is missing on the target assessment

- The resident does not qualify as high-risk AND value of item G1aA or item G1bA is missing on the target assessment

- The resident does not qualify as high-risk and the value of item B1 is missing on the target assessment

Questions to ask regarding residents who triggered this QI/QM:

- Is your facility following the guidance set forth in F314 in the *State Operations Manual*?

- Do definitions provided match those on the MDS and in documentation?

- Is facility using an "at risk" form for assessment?

- Is there documentation of staff training on skin care, pressure points, tissue tolerance, nutrition guidelines, etc.?

- Are there prevention procedure guidelines in the facility policy manual? If so, are they followed and addressed in the care plan?

- Are interventions specific for the resident (such as resident's choices and advance directives) included in the care plan?

- Are pressure ulcers monitored by the physician?

- Are the specific guidelines for documentation set forth in F314 followed by the physician and by nursing staff?

- Are possible infections monitored and pain management measures employed?

- Is the facility familiar with possible other F-tags related to pressure ulcers (such as F501)?

- Pay special attention to residents suffering from dehydration, fecal impaction, urinary tract infections, and weight loss; those with tube feeding; and those whose ADL assistance needs have increased.

- If the resident frequently sits in a chair, is the facility using other measures besides "microshifting" to relieve pressure?

- If the resident refuses prevention measures or treatment, is this documented in the clinical record?

- Ensure that the MDS is filled out correctly.

Post-acute care (PAC) measures

13.1 Short-stay residents with delirium (MDS items B5a–f)

Numerator: Short-stay residents with SNF PPS 14-day assessment with at least one symptom of delirium that is a departure from usual functioning

Denominator: All patients with valid SNF PPS 14-day assessment

Exclusions: Residents satisfying any of the following conditions:

- Residents who are comatose (item B1 = 1) or comatose status is unknown (item B1 value is missing) on the 14-day assessment

- Residents with end-stage renal disease (item J5c is checked) or end-stage disease status is unknown (item J5c value is missing) on the 14-day assessment

- Residents receiving hospice care (item P1ao is checked) or hospice status is unknown (item P1ao status is missing) on the 14-day assessment

- The QM did not trigger (resident was not included in numerator) AND there are missing values on any of the items B5a - B5f on the 14-day assessment

Risk adjustment: Indicator of NO prior residential history preceding the current SNF stay

- Covariate = 1 if there is NO prior residential history indicated by the following condition being satisfied:

  - There is a recent admission assessment AND items AB5a–AB5e are not checked (value 0) AND AB5f is checked (value 1)

- Covariate = 0 if there is prior residential history indicated by either of the following conditions being satisfied:

  - There is a recent admission assessment AND any of the items AB5a–AB5e are checked (value 1) OR AB5f is not checked (value 0)

  - There is no recent admission assessment

Questions to ask regarding residents who triggered this QI/QM:

- Is the delirium caused by medications or medical conditions that causes delirium?
- Is there psychiatry involvement?
- Is delirium causing harm to the resident or others?

13.2 Short-stay residents who had moderate to severe pain (MDS items J2a and J2b)

Numerator: Short-stay residents at SNF PPS 14-day assessment with moderate pain at least daily (item J2a = 2 and item J2b = 2) OR horrible/excruciating pain at any frequency (item J2b = 3)

Denominator: All residents with valid 14-day assessment

Exclusions: Residents satisfying either of the following conditions:

- The values for either item J2a or item J2b are missing on the 14-day assessment
- The values of items J2a and J2b are inconsistent on the 14-day assessment

Questions to ask regarding residents who triggered this QI/QM:

- Is pain medication given prior to treatments/therapy, etc.?
- Is patient taking "as-needed" (PRN) medications on a routine basis?
- Does your facility have a pain assessment and management program?

13.3 Short-stay residents with pressure ulcers (MDS item M2a)

Numerator: Short-stay residents who either:

- Had no pressure ulcers on the SNF PPS 5-day assessment and at least one Stage 1 ulcer on the 14-day assessment OR

- Had a pressure ulcer on the 5-day assessment that failed to improve or worsened on the 14-day assessment

Denominator: All residents with a valid 14-day assessment and a valid preceding 5-day assessment

Exclusions: Residents satisfying either of the following conditions:

- The value for item M2a is missing on the 14-day assessment
- The value for item M2a is missing on the 5-day assessment and item M2a shows presence of pressure sores on the 14-day assessment (item M2a = 1, 2, 3, or 4)

Risk adjustment: Based on the following conditions on the 5-day assessment:

1. Indicator of history of resolved pressure ulcers

    - Covariate = 1 if item M3 = 1
    - Covariate = 0 if item M3 = 0

2. Indicator of requiring limited or more assistance in bed mobility

    - Covariate = 1 if item G1aA = 2, 3, 4, or 8
    - Covariate = 0 if item G1aA = 0 or 1

3. Indicator of bowel incontinence at least once per week

  - Covariate = 1 if item H1a = 2, 3, or 4
  - Covariate = 0 if item H1a = 0 or 1

4. Indicator of diabetes or peripheral vascular disease

  - Covariate = 1 if item I1a check (value 1) OR if item I1j is checked (value 1)
  - Covariate = 0 if item I1a not checked (value 0) AND item I1j is not checked (value 0)

5. Indicator of low Body Mass Index (BMI)

  - Covariate = 1 is BMI $\geq$ 12 and $\leq$ 19
  - Covariate = 0 if BMI > and $\leq$ 40

Questions to ask regarding residents who triggered this QI/QM:

- Was the resident admitted with pressure ulcer? If so, was the ulcer documented/photographed in medical record?

- Was prevention/treatment initiated upon admission?

- Is there documentation of disease processes interfering in ulcer resolution (i.e., surgery, alcoholism, abnormal lab values, malnutrition, etc.?)

Details of the seven QI/QM reports

Details of the seven QI/QM reports

Any facility that wants to make a serious effort at tracking and improving its quality of care will want to access and use the Quality Indicator/Quality Measure (QI/QM) reports it can get online. These are available through the Quality Improvement and Evaluation System (QIES) system you would normally use to transmit your MDS data.

The new reports

There are seven reports in the new system, including:

❑ Facility Characteristics Report

❑ Facility Quality Measure/Indicator Report

❑ Quality Measure/Indicator Monthly Trend Report

❑ Resident Level Quality Measure/Indicator Report: Chronic Care Sample

❑ Resident Listing Report: Chronic Care Sample

❑ Resident Listing Report: Post-Acute Sample

❑ Resident Level Quality Measure/Indicator Report: Post-Acute Sample

Facility Characteristics Report

The Facility Characteristics Report (Figure 3.1) can be used to help identify possible areas for further emphasis or review as part of a survey or a facility's quality assurance and improvement processes.

FIGURE 3.1

Facility Characteristics Report

Facility Name	LISA01	Run Date	06/15/05 15:59:30
City/State	SACRAMENTO, CA	Report Period	12/01/04–05/31/05
Provider Number	855134	Comparison Group	07/01/04–12/31/04
Login/Internal ID	LISA01/1234	Report Version Number	1.07

		Facility		Comparison Group	
	Num	Denom	Observed Percent	State Average	National Average
Gender					
Male	10	24	41.7%	31.2%	31.3%
Female	14	24	58.3%	68.7%	66.7%
Age					
<25 years old	0	24	0.0%	1.0%	0.5%
25-54 years old	0	24	0.0%	5.4%	5.8%
55-64 years old	1	24	4.2%	6.6%	6.7%
65-74 years old	2	24	8.3%	12.5%	13.3%
75-84 years old	8	24	33.3%	31.9%	32.7%
85+ years old	13	24	54.2%	42.4%	40.9%
Payment Source (all that apply)					
Medicaid per diem	0	24	0.0%	50.9%	44.7%
Medicare per diem	10	24	41.7%	29.9%	30.3%
Medicare ancillary Part A	13	24	54.2%	25.3%	18.2%
Medicare ancillary Part B	2	24	8.3%	22.5%	8.4%
Self or family pays full per diem	5	24	20.6%	10.5%	15.1%
Medicaid resident liability or Medicare co-payment	1	24	4.2%	7.9%	10.6%
Private insurance per diem (including co-payment)	4	24	16.7%	10.4%	10.4%
All other per diem	0	24	0.0%	4.0%	3.2%
Diagnostic Characteristics					
Psychiatric diagnosis	1	24	4.2%	11.6%	13.1%
Mental retardation	1	24	4.2%	2.4%	2.7%
Hospice	1	24	4.2%	1.3%	3.2%
Type of Assessment					
Admission assessment	10	24	41,7%	26.4%	31.2%
Annual assessment	3	24	12.5%	12.5%	10.9%
Significant change in status assessment	2	24	8.3%	6.3%	8.4%
Significant correction or prior full assessment	0	24	0.0%	0.0%	0.0%
Quarterly assessment	9	24	37.5%	52.8%	49.4%
Significant correction of prior quarterly assessment	0	24	0.0%	0.0%	0.0%
All other assessment types	0	24	0.0%	0.0%	0.0%
Stability of Conditions					
Conditions/disease make resident unstable	17	24	70.8%	25.4%	41.8%
Acute episode or chronic flareup	0	24	0.0%	11.2%	17.1%
End-stage disease, 6 or fewer months to live	2	24	8.3%	1.7%	2.8%
Discharge Potential					
No discharge potential	12	24	50.0%	66.9%	55.7%
Discharge potential within 30 days	5	24	20.8%	6.9%	10.9%
Discharge potential 30-90 days	4	24	16.7%	7.7%	5.5%
Uncertain discharge potential	2	24	8.3%	15.2%	17.4%

This report contains facility demographic information, including percentages for comparison with state and national averages. By comparing the facility percentages with the state and national average percentages, the user can determine whether the facility's demographic characteristics are unusual.

The report is generated by five submitted assessments, including:

- Admission assessment
- Annual assessment
- Significant change assessment
- Significant change of prior full assessment
- Quarterly assessment or correction of prior quarterly assessment

Facility Quality Measure/Indicator Report

The Facility Quality Measure/Indicator Report, previously known as the Facility Quality Indicator Profile report, shows each QI/QM, the facility percentage, and how the facility compares with other facilities in the state and the nation (Figure 3.2). The comparisons with the state are shown using both percentages and a percentile ranking system.

This report helps you to identify possible areas for further emphasis in facility quality improvement activities or investigation during the survey process. Because the goal is to highlight potential quality of care problems for the facility, this report includes only residents for whom the target assessment is likely to reflect care in the facility. For example, residents with an admission target assessment are excluded from prevalence measures, since conditions present on admission are not likely to reflect care in the facility.

FIGURE 3.2

Facility Quality Measure/Indicator Report

Facility Name	LISA01	Run Date	05/20/05 16:01:28
City/State	SACRAMENTO, CA	Report Period	09/01/04–02/28/05
Provider Number	855134	Comparison Group	07/01/04–12/31/04
Login/Internal ID	LISA01/1234	Report Version Number	1.07

		Facility				Comparison Group		
Measure ID Chronic Care	Domain/Measure Description Measures	Num	Denom	Observed Percent	Adjusted Percent	State Average	National Average	State percentile
	Accidents							
1.1	Incidence of new fractures	1	109	0.9%	-	1.9%	2.1%	29
1.2	Prevalence of falls	5	109	4.6%	-	12.3%	12.9%	8
	Behavioral/Emotional Patterns							
2.1	Residents who have become more depressed or anxious	9	109	8.3%	-	16.1%	15.7%	23
2.2	Prevalence of behavior symptoms affecting others: Overall	16	106	15.1%	-	23.3%	18.9%	26
2.2-HI	Prevalence of behavior symptoms affecting others: High risk	15	86	17.4%	-	26.1%	22.1%	29
2.2-LO	Prevalence of behavior symptoms affecting others: Low risk	1	20	5.0%	-	8.7%	8.1%	49
2.3	Prevalence of symptoms of depression without antidepressant therapy	0	106	0.0%	-	6.7%	5.3%	0
	Clinical Management							
3.1	Use of 9 or more different medications	76	109	69.7%	-	56.2%	60.2%	84
	Cognitive Patterns							
4.1	Incidence of cognitive impairment	1	22	4.5%	-	15.0%	12.3%	23
	Elimination/Incontinence							
5.1	Low-risk residents who lost control of their bowels or bladder	42	67	62.7%	-	47.1%	46.8%	88
5.2	Residents who have/had a catheter inserted and left in their bladder	7	109	6.4%	5.8%	5.2%	7.7%	62
5.3	Prevalence of occasional or frequent bladder or bowel incontinence without a toileting plan	32	33	97.0%	-	54.9%	44.2%	85
5.4	Prevalence of fecal impaction	0	109	0.0%	-	0.2%	0.1%	0
	Infection Control							
6.1	Residents with a urinary tract infections	8	109	7.3%	-	8.5%	9.5%	44
	Nutrition/Eating							
7.1	Residents who lose too much weight	6	90	6.7%	-	10.9%	10.0%	21
7.2	Prevalence of tube feeding	24	109	22.0%	-	9.0%	7.2%	96*
7.3	Prevalence of dehydration	2	109	1.8%	-	0.5%	0.4%	93*
	Pain Management							
8.1	Residents who have moderate to severe pain	13	109	11.9%	9.4%	9.8%	7.8%	61

Note: Dashes represent a value that could not be computed.

FIGURE 3.2

Facility Quality Measure/Indicator Report (cont.)

Measure ID Chronic Care	Domain/Measure Description Measures	Facility				Comparison Group		
		Num	Denom	Observed Percent	Adjusted Percent	State Average	National Average	State percentile
	Physical Functioning							
9.1	Residents whose need for help with daily activities has increased	6	77	7.8%	-	15.6%	17.5%	16
9.2	Residents who spend most of their time in bed or in a chair	29	106	27.4%	-	8.1%	5.5%	98*
9.3	Residents whose ability to move in and around their room got worse	6	52	11.5%	10.1%	14.0%	15.7%	33
9.4	Incidents of decline in ROM	4	105	3.8%	-	8.1%	8.5%	27
	Psychotropic Drug Use							
10.1	Prevalence of antipsychotic use, in the absence of psychotic or related conditions: Overall	18	100	18.0%	-	26.7%	22.0%	20
10.1-HI	Prevalence of antipsychotic use, in the absence of psychotic or related conditions: High risk	7	11	63.6%	-	47.7%	46.0%	83
10.1-LO	Prevalence of antipsychotic use, in the absence of psychotic or related conditions: Low risk	11	86	12.8%	-	22.2%	18.1%	18
10.2	Prevalence of antianxiety/ hypnotic use	20	100	20.0%	-	18.6%	18.8%	58
10.3	Prevalence of hypnotic use more than two times in the last week	3	109	2.8%	-	3.8%	4.1%	47
	Quality of Life							
11.1	Residents who were physically restrained	8	109	7.3%	-	9.8%	7.1%	40
11.2	Prevalence of little or no activity	65	106	61.3%	-	10.5%	9.2%	99*
	Skin Care							
12.1	High-risk residents with pressure ulcers	13	75	17.3%	-	17.1%	15.2%	58
12.2	Low-risk resident with pressure ulcers	1	34	2.9%	-	2.9%	3.4%	64*
	Post-Acute Care (PAC) Measures							
13.1	Short-stay residents with delirium	5	86	5.8%	5.2%	4.8%	3.4%	69
13.2	Short-stay residents who had moderate to severe pain	44	86	51.2%	-	23.5%	23.7%	92*
13.3	Short-stay residents with pressure ulcers	20	83	24.1%	23.4%	19.7%	18.8%	67

Note: Dashes represent a value that could not be computed.

Facility Section

All of the facility results in this column are for the user-selected *Report Period* given in the report header.

The first column is *Num*. This represents the number of residents who triggered the QI/QM (i.e., the people who "have" the QI/QM). For the purposes of calculating the facility percentage, it is the numerator.

The second column is *Denom*. This is the number of people in the facility who "could have" the QI/QM. For the purposes of calculating facility percentage, it is the denominator.

For some measures, the number of cases in the denominator will be equal to the current number of chronic care or post-acute care residents in the facility. For other measures, the denominator will be limited to a specific subgroup of residents who "could have" triggered the QI/QM.

The third column is the *Observed Percent*. This column shows the percentage of residents who could have the QI/QM and actually triggered it. For instance, if 60 people could trigger a measure (*Denom* column) and 30 people actually did trigger it (*Num* column), the facility *Observed Percent* column would be 50%.

The fourth column is the *Adjusted Percent*. The *Adjusted Percent* applies a mathematical model that takes other health characteristics of the resident and the national percent for the measure into account and adjusts the observed percent accordingly. This methodology is applied to only a subset of measures; therefore the *Adjusted Percent* is reported only for those measures (e.g., measure 5.2).

Comparison Group Section

The statistics reported in the *Comparison Group* section in the body of the report are based upon QI/QM calculations that are performed for every facility in your state and in the nation. These calculations are performed on a monthly basis.

When you request a report, the reporting software offers the most recent comparison period as a default (you may change this and select an earlier comparison group period if you wish). The exact comparison group period that was used to produce the report is indicated in the header of the report next to the *Comparison Group* title.

The first column is the *State Average*. This column shows the average statewide percentage for the QM for comparison with the facility. It represents the simple average of the observed percentages (or the adjusted percentages, for risk-adjusted measures) across all facilities in your state. This column can be very helpful in determining whether a facility is substantially above or below the statewide percentage. Such facilities are called "outliers," meaning their percentages are unusual with respect to the rest of the state.

The second column is the *National Average*. This column is new for the report and shows the average observed or adjusted percentage for the measure for all facilities in the nation. Again, this column allows comparisons with the facility percent.

The third column is the *State Percentile*. This column ranks facilities relative to other facilities in the state on each measure. The higher the ranking, the more likely the measure needs to be reviewed as part of the facility quality improvement process or emphasized on the survey. The values in this column represent the percent of facilities in the state that are at or below the observed (or adjusted) percentage for your facility.

For example, if your facility is at the 85th percentile for a measure, it means that 85% of the facilities in the state have an observed (or adjusted) percentage that is at or below your facility's percentage.

Some of the values in the *State Percentile* column may be followed by an asterisk. The asterisk identifies those measures that have crossed an investigative threshold (those that have been "flagged"). This column identifies those measures where the facility's ranking is high enough that it should be investigated or emphasized on the survey or in any internal quality improvement initiative. It means that this facility's performance on this particular QM is higher than some critical value, and there is a possible concern for the quality of care. It is an area to highlight for investigation or emphasis during offsite survey preparation or to choose for review in the facility quality assurance or quality improvement processes. QI/QMs at or above the 90th percentile in this column will be designated by an asterisk (*). All sentinel health event measures (5.4 Prevalence of Fecal Impaction, 7.3 Prevalence of Dehydration, and 12.2 Prevalence of Stage 1–4 Pressure Ulcers-Low Risk) with any triggering cases (a numerator larger than zero) will also be designated by an asterisk (*).

What does this report say about a facility's care?

High QI/QM scores may or may not reflect poor care. For instance, a facility that specializes in wound care may have a high percentile ranking for pressure ulcers. A facility with high behavior scores may specialize in dementia care. Therefore, prior to judging care based on quality indicators that are higher than those of other facilities, it is important to find out if the facility specializes in care that would cause these quality indicators to be high.

Indicators may also impact each other. For example, a facility that gives more psychotropic medications may experience a higher percentile ranking of falls. The fall may contribute to a higher percentile ranking of fractures. If a resident is incontinent without a toileting plan and has significant weight loss, he or she may be more likely to develop a pressure ulcer. Combining review of the quality indicator report and the past State Survey results will give a clearer indication of care.

Quality Measure/Indicator Monthly Trend Report

This new report shows a facility's monthly scores on any single QI/QM measure. The months displayed are based upon a time period selected by the user. For each month, the report displays the facility's score as well as the average score for the facility's state and for the nation. The scores for each month represent QI/QM calculations for the six-month target period ending with that month.

The scores are observed QI/QM percentages for most measures but adjusted QI/QM percentages for risk-adjusted measures. The data are displayed in both graphical and tabular form, allowing the user to determine whether the facility's scores are increasing or decreasing over time and how those scores compare with state and national averages.

The report title indicates the QI/QM measure being reported. The report header includes the report period selected by the user. In the graph, the red line shows the facility's QI/QM percentage for each month (six-month target period ending with that month). The green and blue lines are the corresponding national and state percentages for each target period. The Y-axis title will indicate whether the observed percent or adjusted percent is being reported for this measure.

The same data are also presented in the table below the graph. The *report period* columns give the six-month report period for each set of facility, state, and national scores. For each report period, the facility columns give the facility numerator count in the *Num* column, the facility denominator count in the *Den* column, and facility observed percentage in the *Obs Pcnt* column. If an adjusted QI/QM is reported, the facility adjusted percentage would be reported and the column would be labeled *Adj Pcnt* rather than *Obs Pcnt*. Finally, for each report period, the *Comparison Group* columns give the average observed (or adjusted) *state* and *national* percentages for the measure.

FIGURE 3.3

Quality Measure/Indicator: Monthly Trend Report

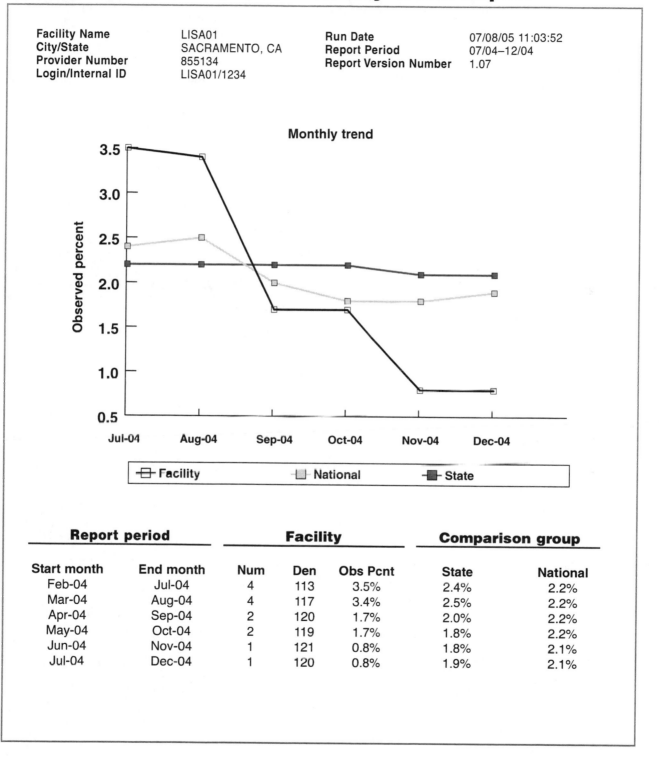

Facility Name	LISA01	Run Date	07/08/05 11:03:52
City/State	SACRAMENTO, CA	Report Period	07/04–12/04
Provider Number	855134	Report Version Number	1.07
Login/Internal ID	LISA01/1234		

Monthly trend

Report period		Facility			Comparison group	
Start month	End month	Num	Den	Obs Pcnt	State	National
Feb-04	Jul-04	4	113	3.5%	2.4%	2.2%
Mar-04	Aug-04	4	117	3.4%	2.5%	2.2%
Apr-04	Sep-04	2	120	1.7%	2.0%	2.2%
May-04	Oct-04	2	119	1.7%	1.8%	2.2%
Jun-04	Nov-04	1	121	0.8%	1.8%	2.1%
Jul-04	Dec-04	1	120	0.8%	1.9%	2.1%

Resident Level Quality Measure/Indicator Report: Chronic Care Sample

This report contains data for those residents who are included in the chronic care sample because they have an OBRA assessment (admission, quarterly, annual, significant change, or significant correction assessment) in the user-selected *Report Period* given in the report header (Figure 3.4). It is possible for residents to be included in both the chronic care and post-acute care samples if they have qualifying OBRA and post-acute assessments during the target period.

In this report, residents are listed in two groups: active residents and discharged residents (residents whose last MDS record during the target period was a discharge). Residents are listed in alphabetical order within each of these two groups. The report identifies each resident by his or her resident internal ID and name. The primary reason for assessment (AA8a) for the selected OBRA target assessment is also listed.

Following the identifying information, the report contains columns for each QI/QM. An X appears in the QI/QM column when the resident triggers a measure (i.e., is included in the numerator for that measure). The last column in each row displays a count of the number of measures that were triggered for the resident.

Recall that residents with admission target assessments are excluded from the observed (or adjusted) facility percentages for prevalence measures on the previous report (Facility Quality Measure/Indicator Report). This exclusion ensures that facility percentages do not include residents with conditions present on admission, conditions that do not reflect care in the facility. However, in the present report (Resident Level Quality Measure/Indicator Report: Chronic Care Sample), all chronic care residents are listed regardless of whether the target assessment is an admission assessment or not. The triggering status of these residents is listed for all chronic care measures (including prevalence measures).

The Resident Level Quality Measure/Indicator Report can be used in two ways. First, it can be used to identify the residents that trigger a particular QI/QM (by scanning a column of interest and looking for the residents with an X). Second, it can be used to identify residents who trigger multiple QI/QM measures. Such residents may merit special consideration or more intensive review.

FIGURE 3.4

Resident Level Quality Measure/Indicator Report: Chronic Care Sample

Facility Name LISA01
City/State SACRAMENTO, CA
Provider Number 855134
Login/Internal ID LISA01/1234

Run Date 08/15/05 15:59:30
Report Period 12/01/04–05/31/05
Report Version Number 1.07

Resident Int ID	Resident name	AA8a	Accid: New tract	Accid: Falls	Behav: Depression	Behav: Problem Behavior (Hi/Lo)	Behav: Dprs No Tx	ClinCog: 9+ Meds	ClinCog: Cog Impair	Elim: Bwl/Blad Incont (Lo)	Elim: Cath Insert	Elim: Incont No TP	Elim: Fecal Impct	Infct: UTIs	Nutrit: Wt. Loss	Nutrit: Tube Feed	Nutrit: Dhyd	Pain: Mod/Sevr Pain	Phys: ADL Help Incrs	Phys: Most Time Chair	Phys: Move Ability Wrse	Phys: Declin ROM	Psych: Antipsy w/o psychotic condition (Hi/Lo)	Psych: Anti-anx/Hpnot	Psych: Hpnot 2x Week	QualLife: Phys Restrn	QualLife: Little Activ	Skin: Pressure Ulcers (Hi/Lo)	Count
Active Residents																													
999999	Doe, Jane	D2						X									X												2
999999	Doe, Jane	D5		X				X						X														X	5
999999	Doe, Jane	D5			X			X	X										X											2
999999	Doe, Jane	D3						X	X	X					X															4
999999	Doe, Jane	D2		X		X		X		X									X											3
999999	Doe, Jane	D5						X							X														X	1
999999	Doe, Jane	D1								X				X				X											X	5
999999	Doe, Jane	D1								X													X							2
999999	Doe, Jane	D1		X				X										X					X						X	3
999999	Doe, Jane	D1						X																X	X				X	5
999999	Doe, Jane	D1						X																X	X					2
999999	Doe, Jane	D5																												0
999999	Doe, Jane	D5								X				X																2
999999	Doe, Jane	D5		X										X								X								2
999999	Doe, Jane	D2						X																						1
999999	Doe, Jane	D1								X									X				X						X	2
999999	Doe, Jane	D3		X	X			X												X										4
999999	Doe, Jane	D1						X											X		X	X								2
999999	Doe, Jane	D1			X			X							X				X											4
999999	Doe, Jane	D5		X	X																								X	2
999999	Doe, Jane	D5			X													X						X	X				X	5
Discharged Residents																													
999999	Doe, Jane	D1																												4

Note: x=triggered, blank=not triggered or excluded.

Resident Listing Report: Chronic Care Sample

The Resident Listing Report: Chronic Care Sample lists those residents who are included in the chronic care sample, because they have an OBRA admission, quarterly, annual, significant change, or significant correction assessment in the target period (Figure 3.5). The residents listed in this report match those in the chronic care Resident Level Quality Measure/Quality Indicator Report. Like that report, the Resident Listing Report divides residents into two groups: active and discharged. Residents are listed alphabetically within each of those groups. The purpose of the Resident Listing Report is to supply supplementary information about the residents in the chronic care sample.

The first column, *Resident Int Id* (resident internal ID), displays the ID that is assigned when the assessment record is submitted to the state database. It can be used to link data on the Resident Listing Report with data on the Resident Level Quality Measure/Indicator Report.

The *Resident Name* column displays the resident's last name and first name. The *Gender* column displays the resident's gender. The DOB column contains the resident's birth date and the *Room No* column displays his or her room number.

Two columns display the information about the selected assessments, one for the *Target Assessment* and one for the *Prior Assessment*. Sub-columns for the target and prior assessments are *A3a* (assessment reference date) and *AA8a/AA8b* (primary and special reason for assessment).

The last column displayed on this report is the *Discharge Date*. This field is blank for active residents, and shows the most recent discharge date for residents who were discharged at the end of the target period. Note that discharges occurring before the target assessment reference date are not shown.

FIGURE 3.5

Resident Listing Report: Chronic Care Sample

Facility Name	LISA01	Run Date	01/12/2005 12:44:22
City/State	SACRAMENTO, CA	Report Period	10/01/2003–03/31/2004
Provider Number	855134	Report Version Number	1.07
Login/Internal ID	LISA01/1234		

					Target assessment		Prior assessment		
Resident Int Id	Resident name	Gender	DOB	Room No.	A3a	AA8a/AA8b	A3a	AA8a/AA8b	Discharge date
Active Residents									
999999	Doe, John	M	09/07/1921	0362	02/25/2004	05/6	12/08/2003	01/1	
999999	Doe, John	M	06/10/1915	362-1	03/17/2004	05/6	12/30/2003	01/1	
999999	Doe, John	M	02/06/1901	360-2	03/17/2004	05/6	12/24/2003	01/1	
999999	Doe, John	M	01/25/1902	3501	03/24/2004	05/6	13/30/2003	01/1	
999999	Doe, John	M	04/13/1903	0349	03/16/2004	01/1		/	
999999	Doe, John	M	07/30/1916	0340	02/21/2004	01/1		/	
999999	Doe, John	M	09/03/1911	0348	03/05/2004	01/1		/	
999999	Doe, John	M	06/03/1911	3502	01/21/2004	05/6	10/29/2003	05/6	
999999	Doe, John	F	08/23/1923	0348	12/22/2003	01/1		/	
999999	Doe, John	M	01/31/1925	343	02/25/2004	05/6	12/08/2003	05/6	
999999	Doe, John	M	10/09/1921	0357	03/16/2004	01/1		/	
999999	Doe, John	M	11/26/1916	362-2	01/07/2004	05/6	10/18/2003	01/6	
999999	Doe, John	M	02/08/1908	0341	03/10/2004	05/6	12/12/2003	01/1	
999999	Doe, John	M	09/17/1911	346	02/04/2004	05/6	11/11/2003	02/6	
999999	Doe, John	M	11/04/1913	0354	03/25/2004	01/1		/	
Discharged Residents									
999999	Doe, John	M	09/19/1917	0349	01/13/2004	01/1	11/21/2003	01/1	01/26/2004
999999	Doe, John	M	06/15/1925	0357	03/09/2004	01/1		/	03/14/2004
999999	Doe, John	M	01/27/1929	0359	12/29/2003	01/1		/	01/23/2004
999999	Doe, John	M	09/05/1910	0354	11/25/2003	01/1		/	12/06/2003
999999	Doe, John	M	03/25/1908	350-1	01/21/2004	05/6	10/29/2003	05/6	03/24/2004
999999	Doe, John	M	02/16/1927	0357	01/16/2004	01/1		/	02/11/2004
999999	Doe, John	M	06/29/1910	357	10/06/2003	02/6	07/16/2003	05/6	01/09/2004
999999	Doe, John	F	10/01/1916	0349	03/10/2004	01/1		/	03/15/2004
999999	Doe, John	M	06/02/1917	0340	11/07/2003	01/1		/	11/13/2003
999999	Doe, John	F	12/09/1918	0348	12/02/2003	01/1		/	12/17/2003
999999	Doe, John	M	09/15/1920	0348	01/30/2004	01/1		/	02/09/2004
999999	Doe, John	M	09/08/1913	0349	12/30/2003	01/1		/	01/08/2004
999999	Doe, John	F	10/03/1922	0354	11/13/2003	01/1		/	11/20/2003
999999	Doe, John	M	11/06/1926	0359	02/21/2004	01/1		/	02/25/2004
999999	Doe, John	F	06/20/1920	0349	12/16/2003	01/1		/	12/30/2003
999999	Doe, John	M	04/24/1918	0357	02/25/2004	01/1		/	03/08/2004
999999	Doe, John	M	03/23/1925	0359	03/16/2004	01/1		/	03/26/2004
999999	Doe, John	M	06/18/1916	0360	11/12/2003	01/1		/	12/01/2003
999999	Doe, John	M	09/21/1910	0360	12/12/2003	01/1		/	12/22/2003
999999	Doe, John	M	04/19/1916	0362	10/27/2003	01/1		/	11/06/2003
999999	Doe, John	M	03/26/1925	0349	02/09/2004	01/1		/	02/15/2004
999999	Doe, John	M	01/10/1917	0349	10/23/2003	01/1		/	12/12/2003
999999	Doe, John	M	12/17/1923	0348	02/17/2004	01/1		/	02/26/2004
999999	Doe, John	M	07/12/1915	0360	10/30/2003	01/1		/	11/10/2003
999999	Doe, John	M	02/19/1926	0354	12/13/2003	01/1		/	12/17/2003
999999	Doe, John	F	12/11/1915	0346	01/16/2004	01/1	09/15/2003	01/1	01/22/2004
999999	Doe, John	M	06/27/1926	0354	12/18/2003	01/1		/	12/29/2003
999999	Doe, John	F	06/26/1917	0354	10/30/2003	01/1		/	11/12/2003

Resident Level Quality Measure/Indicator Report: Post-Acute Care Sample

This new report (Figure 3.6) parallels the chronic care report described above (Figure 3.5). It contains data for residents who are in the post-acute care sample (who had a 14-day SNF PPS assessment during the target period). In all other respects, it parallels the chronic care report.

FIGURE 3.6

Resident Level Quality Measure/Indicator Report: Post-Acute Care Sample

Facility Name	LISA01	
City/State	SACRAMENTO, CA	
Provider Number	855134	
Login/Internal ID	LISA01/1234	

Run Date	08/15/05 15:59:30
Report Period	12/01/04–05/31/05
Report Version Number	1.07

Resident Int ID	Resident name	Delrm	Mod/Sevr Pain	Press Ulcer	Count
Active Residents					
999999	Doe, Jane			X	1
999999	Doe, Jane				0
999999	Doe, Jane				0
999999	Doe, Jane		X	X	2
999999	Doe, John			X	1
999999	Doe, John				0
999999	Doe, John				0
999999	Doe, John				0
Discharged Residents					
999999	Doe, Jane		X	X	2
999999	Doe, Jane		X		1
999999	Doe, John				0
999999	Doe, John				0

Note: x=triggered, blank=not triggered or excluded.

Resident Listing Report: Post-Acute Care Sample

This new report (Figure 3.7). parallels the chronic care Resident Listing report described above. It lists the residents who are in the post-acute care sample (who had a 14-day SNF PPS assessment during the target period). In all other respects, it parallels the chronic care report.

FIGURE 3.7

Resident Listing Report: Post-Acute Care Sample

Facility Name	LISA01	Run Date	01/12/2005 12:23:04
City/State	SACRAMENTO, CA	Report Period	10/01/2003–03/31/2004
Provider Number	855134	Report Version Number	1.07
Login/Internal ID	LISA01/1234		

Resident Int Id	Resident name	Gender	DOB	Room No.	Target assessment A3a	Target assessment AA8a/ AA8b	Prior assessment A3a	Prior assessment AA8a/ AA8b	Discharge date
Active Residents									
999999	Doe, John	M	09/07/1921	0362	12/13/2003	00/7	12/03/2003	01/1	
999999	Doe, John	M	01/25/1902	0354	01/09/2004	00/7	12/30/2003	01/1	
999999	Doe, John	M	07/30/1916	0359	03/02/2004	00/7	02/21/2004	01/1	
999999	Doe, John	M	09/03/1911	0348	03/15/2004	00/7	03/05/2004	01/1	
999999	Doe, John	M	10/09/1921	0357	03/26/2004	00/7	03/16/2004	01/1	
Discharged Residents									
999999	Doe, John	M	01/27/1929	0359	01/08/2004	00/7	12/29/2003	01/1	01/23/2004
999999	Doe, John	M	09/05/1910	0354	12/05/2003	00/7	11/25/2003	01/1	12/09/2003
999999	Doe, John	M	02/16/1927	0357	01/26/2004	00/7	01/16/2004	01/1	02/11/2004
999999	Doe, John	F	12/09/1918	0348	12/12/2003	00/7	12/02/2003	01/1	12/17/2003
999999	Doe, John	M	08/18/1916	0360	11/22/2003	00/7	11/12/2003	01/1	12/01/2003
999999	Doe, John	M	01/10/1917	0349	11/04/2003	00/7	10/23/2003	01/1	12/12/2003
999999	Doc, John	M	06/28/1906	0348	11/03/2003	00/7	10/24/2003	01/1	11/21/2003
999999	Doe, John	M	03/19/1909	0359	01/29/2004	00/7	01/19/2004	01/1	02/06/2004

Accessing the reports

The QI/QM reports arrive in your electronic mailbox on a quarterly basis as a folder in the Quality Improvement and Evaluation System (QIES).

To pull up your QI/QM information, follow these steps:

1. Start your MDS computer system. "Welcome to the CMS MDS System" will appear on the first screen.

2. Click on the icon for CASPER reports in the online reports section.

3. Go to the CASPER login page by clicking on "Connect to MDS Online reports."

4. Enter the same user identification and password that you would use to submit your MDS data to the state.

5. The next screen will contain a box in the upper left-hand corner. In the lower right-hand corner of the box, click on "login," which will bring you to the CASPER homepage.

6. Go to the top menu bar and click on the "folders" tab.

7. Go to the heading that reads "folders, my inbox." Click on the asterisk before that heading.

Conclusion:
Ensuring quality care

Conclusion: Ensuring quality care

The Quality Indicators/Quality Measures: A road map for providing optimum care

The QI/QMs serve as a guide to determine whether quality care is present. However, if a particular indicator does not flag, that does not necessarily guarantee that quality care is provided in that area. Therefore, nursing facilities should not only monitor QI/QM reports but also consider internal quality improvement activities.

How can you ensure quality care in your facility? Making sure that you meet regulatory requirements for each of the QI/QMs should start you off in the right direction. Instead of meeting basic required standards, nursing facilities should seek to exceed and improve upon CMS' quality standards.

The QI/QMs are a guideline to help facilities focus on potential areas for quality improvement actions. However, facilities should not stop there. For example, if the prevalence of daily physical restraints is below the percentile rank that would cause concern but is still too high in the facility's judgment, the facility should establish restraint reduction programs. Using the MDS data to direct their efforts, staff can investigate if any one section of the nursing home uses more restraints than other sections, if the restraints are used more on certain shifts, or if certain staff members apply restraints more freely than others. As staff conducts further investigation of each of these areas, they may hone in on potential solutions or the implementation of systems that may continue to decrease restraint use.

Eliciting ideas from all staff members—especially nursing assistants, who typically have the most direct contact with residents—can yield excellent recommendations for improvement in all the quality domains.

The importance of proactive care planning

Accurate assessment and completion of the MDS are only two aspects of continuing quality care. The quality indicator information obtained from the MDS assessments begins the process for determining quality, but it cannot end there.

Based on careful scrutiny of the assessment data and QI/QMs that have flagged, facilities must make appropriate plans to maintain or improve quality of care and implement them. Specific ideas and methods determined to be important and beneficial need to be put in place. Finally, evaluation of the effectiveness of the action or plan should reveal the need for revisions or adjustments.

The QI/QMs provide a starting point for defining and measuring what it means to deliver quality care to residents. However, they provide only one piece of the puzzle. In the final analysis, what constitutes "quality" care is a highly personal and subjective matter and depends on the individuals involved. The QI/QMs can point a facility in the proper direction and provide the framework for proper care planning. However, the continual planning, implementation, and evaluation process should be individualized for each facility, based on the particular needs of the residents. A quality improvement plan that works extremely well in one nursing home may be completely wrong for another facility. Each facility should implement plans for quality improvement through an in-depth analysis of its unique quality concerns.

Although these QI/QMs were designed as a tool to measure quality more objectively, undoubtedly more changes and additions to the system will arise. Will an ideal, comprehensive system guaranteed to completely measure quality ever be developed? Probably not. Quality is a subjective concept: although one resident at a long-term care facility may be pleased with the level of service provided, the resident in the next room may perceive a lack of quality despite receiving identical services.

Healthcare providers should consider all of the varying perceptions and ideas about quality and attempt to provide both required and requested healthcare services for all residents.

Most caretakers entered the healthcare field because they wanted to take good care of people and promote health. Similarly, providing optimum care for residents is the main goal of every long-term care facility. Quality is an abstract concept; but this healthcare mission—to provide the best possible care—is the common theme. Maintaining and promoting the dignity and independence of every resident are paramount to achieving this goal. Through dedication to the commitment of ensuring quality care, the healthcare industry can use the information from the quality indicators to rise to an even higher level of success in patient care.

The merged quality indicator/quality measure crosschecker

The merged quality indicator/ quality measure crosschecker

CMS merged the quality indicators (QI) and quality measures (QM) it uses for survey purposes into one group of indicators and measures. They are derived from information coded on the MDS. The chart starting on the next page lists them and the corresponding MDS items used to calculate the QI/QMs.

Quality indicators		Corresponding MDS items
1.1	Incidence of new fractures	**J4c:** Hip fracture in last 180 days (checked on current MDS and not on previous MDS); or **J4d:** Other fracture in last 180 days (checked on current MDS and not on previous MDS)
1.2	Prevalence of falls	**J4a:** Fell in past 30 days (item is checked)
2.1	Residents who have become more depressed or anxious	**E1:** Indicators of depression, anxiety, and sad mood are worse than the previous assessment. Includes E1a (negative statements), E1c (repetitive verbalizations), E1e (self deprecation), E1f (unrealistic fears), E1g (recurrent statements that something terrible will happen), E1h (repetitive health complaints), E1m (crying, tearfulness), E1n (repetitive physical movements), and E2 (depressed or anxious mood not easily altered). Also includes K4c, leaves food uneaten, on target or last full assessment that is a quarterly where the state quarterly assessment does not include item K4c.
2.2-HI	Prevalence of behavior symptoms affecting others, high-risk	**E4b Box A:** Verbally abusive within last seven days; or **E4c Box A:** Physically abusive within last seven days; or **E4d Box A:** Socially inappropriate/disruptive within last seven days Risk adjustment for high-risk: Cognitive impairment in item B4, daily decision-making, and item B2a indicates short-term memory problems or; Item I3 indicates psychotic disorders in the range of ICD-9-CM codes from 295, 297, or 298 series or I1gg, schizophrenia is checked on target or last full assessment that is a quarterly where the state quarterly assessment does not include item I1gg.
2.2-LO	Prevalence of behavior symptoms affecting others, low-risk	**E4bA:** Verbally abusive within last seven days; or **E4cA:** Physically abusive within last seven days; or **E4dA:** Socially inappropriate/disruptive within past seven days Risk adjustment for low-risk: includes all residents who are not high-risk.
2.3	Prevalence of symptoms of depression without antide-pressant therapy	**O4c:** Antidepressant coded 0 and **E2:** Mood persistence coded 1 or 2 and at least two of the following: • Distress, as found in item E1a (negative statements) • Agitation or withdrawal, as found in items E1n (repetitive physical movements), E4eA (resists care), E1o (withdrawal from activity), or E1p (reduced social activity)

Quality indicators		Corresponding MDS items
		• Depression affecting sleep, as found in E1j (unpleasant mood in morning), N1d (no time awake); OR one or none of these three items is checked: N1a (awake in morning), N1b (awake in afternoon), or N1c (awake in evening); and B1 (comatose) not coded 0 • Suicidal or recurrent thoughts of death, as found in item E1g • Weight loss, as found in item K3a
3.1	Use of nine or more different medications	**O1:** Number of medications coded 9 or higher
4.1	Incidence of cognitive impairment	**B4:** Cognitive skills for daily decision-making coded 1, 2, or 3, and not on previous MDS **B2a:** Short-term memory coded 1 and not on previous MDS
5.1	Low-risk residents who lost control of their bowels or bladder	**H1a:** Bowel incontinence coded 3 or 4; or **H2a:** Bladder incontinence coded 3 or 4 Exclusions include those who have a severe cognitive impairment indicated by B4 coded 3 and B2a=1 or are totally dependent in activities of daily living (ADL), evidenced by G1aA coded 4 or 8, G1bA coded 4 or 8, and G1eA coded 4 or 8. Also excludes those who are comatose, have an indwelling catheter, or an ostomy.
5.2	Residents who have/had a catheter inserted and left in their bladder	**H3d:** Indwelling catheter. Covariates consider bowel incontinence and stage 3–4 pressure ulcers.
5.3	Prevalence of occasional or frequent bladder or bowel incontinence without a toileting plan	**H1b:** Bladder incontinence coded 2 or 3; or **H1a:** Bowel incontinence coded 2 or 3; and Neither H3a, any scheduled toileting program, nor H3b, bladder retraining program, is checked
5.4	Prevalence of fecal impaction	**H2d:** Fecal impaction
6.1	Residents with a urinary tract infection (UTI)	**I2j:** UTI in past 30 days
7.1	Residents who lose too much weight	**K3a:** Weight loss coded 1 An exclusion for this item is if P1ao, hospice care, is checked.

Quality indicators	Corresponding MDS items
7.2 Prevalence of tube feeding	**K5b:** Feeding tube checked
7.3 Prevalence of dehydration	**J1c:** Dehydrated (output exceeds input) is coded or **I3:** Contains ICD-9 code 276.5 denoting dehydration
8.1 Residents who have moderate to severe pain	**J2a:** Moderate pain at least daily coded 2; and **J2b:** Horrible/excruciating pain coded 2; or **J2b:** Horrible/excruciating pain at any frequency coded 3 Covariates consider item B4, cognitive skills for daily decision-making.
9.1 Residents whose need for help with daily activities has increased	**G1aA:** Bed mobility self-performance **G1bA:** Transfer self-performance **G1hA:** Eating self-performance **G1iA:** Toilet use self-performance This measures a decline in ADL function over two periods—the current and prior MDS. Include resident if MDS codes indicate a one-level decline in at least two of the above ADLs; or if a two-level decline in one of them. Exclusions include when item B1, comatose, J5c, end-stage disease, or P1ao, hospice care, is checked.
9.2 Residents who spend most of their time in bed or a chair	**G6a:** Bedfast all or most of the time is checked The exclusion is item B1, comatose, is checked.
9.3 Residents whose ability to move in and around their rooms got worse	**G1eA:** Locomotion on unit worsened from previous assessment Covariates include J4a, recent falls, J4b, accidents, G1hA, eating, and G1iA, toileting.
9.4 Incidence of decline in range of motion (ROM)	**G4aA:** Neck ROM **G4bA:** Arm ROM **G4cA:** Hand ROM **G4dA:** Leg ROM **G4eA:** Foot ROM **G4fA:** Other ROM Sum total of 0, 1, and 2 for above six areas of ROM on current MDS greater than on previous MDS. Exclusions include residents with maximal loss of ROM on previous assessment in items G4a–f, box A.

Quality indicators	Corresponding MDS items
10.1-HI Prevalence of antipsychotic use, in the absence of psychotic or related conditions, high-risk	**O4a:** Antipsychotic coded 1 or above Exclusions for this measure include I1gg, schizophrenia, J1i, hallucinations, and ICD-9 codes in item I3 that denote psychotic disorders, Tourette's, or Huntington's disease. High-risk residents comprise those with cognitive impairment and behavior problems, where item B4 is greater than 0, B2a indicates short-term memory problems, and the resident experiences one or more behavior problem daily regarding item E4bA, verbal abuse, E4cA, physical abuse, or E4dA, socially inappropriate or disruptive behavior.
10.1-LO Prevalence of antipsychotic use, in the absence of psychotic or related conditions, low-risk	**O4a:** Antipsychotic coded 1 or above Exclusions for this measure include I1gg, schizophrenia, J1i, hallucinations, and ICD-9 codes in item I3 that denote psychotic disorders, Tourette's, or Huntington's disease. Low-risk residents include any who do not fall into the high-risk group.
10.2 Prevalence of antianxiety/ hypnotic use	**O4b:** Antianxiety coded 1 or above; or **O4d:** Hypnotic coded 1 or above Exclusions for this measure include I1gg, schizophrenia, J1i, hallucinations, and ICD-9 codes in item I3 that denote psychotic disorders, Tourette's, or Huntington's disease.
10.3 Prevalence of hypnotic use more than two times in last week	**O4d:** Hypnotic coded 3 or above
11.1 Residents who were physically restrained	**P4c:** Trunk restraint coded 2; or **P4d:** Limb restraint coded 2; or **P4e:** Chair prevents rising coded 2
11.2 Prevalence of little or no activity	**N2:** Average time involved in activities coded 2 or 3 for little or no activity An exclusion applies to residents for whom B1 is coded 1 for comatose.

Quality indicators	Corresponding MDS items
12.1 High-risk residents with pressure ulcers	**M2a:** Pressure ulcers coded 1 or greater; or **I3:** Contains ICD-9 code 707.0 High-risk residents include those who bed mobility or transfer abilities are coded 3 in items G1aA or G1bA, those who are coded as comatose in item B1, or those whose assessments reflect an ICD-9 code for malnutrition in item I3.
12.2 Low-risk residents with pressure ulcers	**M2a:** Pressure ulcers coded 1 or greater; or **I3:** Contains ICD-9 code 707.0 Low-risk residents are those who do not satisfy the high-risk conditions listed above.
13.1 Short-stay residents with delirium	**B5a–f:** Indicators or delirium—periodic disordered thinking/awareness coded 2 or higher in one or more fields on the 14-day PPS MDS. Exclusions include when item B1, comatose, J5c, end-stage disease, or P1ao, hospice care, is checked. Covariates consider whether the resident had a prior residential history.
13.2 Short-stay residents who had moderate to severe pain	**J2a:** Moderate pain at least daily coded 2; or **J2b:** Horrible/excruciating pain at any frequency coded 3 on the 14-day PPS MDS
13.3 Short-stay residents with pressure ulcers	**M2a:** Pressure ulcers coded on the 14-day PPS MDS and not on the admission MDS or the pressure ulcer worsened or failed to improve between the admission MDS and the 14-day assessment Covariates consider a history of resolved pressure ulcers, limited bed mobility, bowel incontinence, diabetes, peripheral vascular disease, and low body-mass index.

Quality improvement forms

Quality improvement forms

The following forms will help you better manage and track your quality improvement efforts:

- Figure B.1: Restraint elimination/reduction assessment
- Figure B.2: Restraint needs assessment
- Figure B.3: Incident/accident form
- Figure B.4: Pain management assessment form
- Figure B.5: Assessment for bowel and bladder management
- Figure B.6: Pressure ulcer prevention measures
- Figure B.7: Fall assessment tool

FIGURE B.1

Restraint elimination/reduction assessment

Resident Name: _____ Room/Unit #: _____ MD: _____

Assessment date: _____

1. Is resident on facility fall prevention program? _____Y   _____N
2. Present restraint used: _____
3. Resident candidate for restraint reduction or elimination: _____Y   _____N
4. If "yes," date program to start _____/_____/_____
5. If "no," reason: _____
6. Less restrictive measures to be used/attempted: _____
7. Additional comments: _____
8. Team signatures/title: _____ _____

    _____ _____

Assessment date: _____

1. Is resident on facility fall prevention program? _____Y   _____N
2. Present restraint used:_____
3. Resident candidate for restraint reduction or elimination: _____Y   _____N
4. If "yes," date program to start _____/_____/_____
5. If "no," reason: _____
6. Less restrictive measures to be used/attempted: _____
7. Additional comments: _____
8. Team signatures/title: _____ _____

    _____ _____

Assessment date:_____

1. Is resident on facility fall prevention program? _____Y   _____N
2. Present restraint used: _____
3. Resident candidate for restraint reduction or elimination: _____Y   _____N
4. If "yes," date program to start _____/_____/_____
5. If "no," reason: _____
6. Less restrictive measures to be used/attempted: _____
7. Additional comments: _____
8. Team signatures/title: _____ _____

    _____ _____

FIGURE B.2

Restraint needs assessment

1. **Determine factors that may require restraint use, such as:**

   ❑ History of falls that hasn't improved despite interventions
   ❑ Destructive, agitated behavior that impedes safety despite interventions; resistance to treatment/meds/nourishment
   ❑ Gait disturbance
   ❑ Confusion
   ❑ Impaired cognition; unable to follow safety cues and direction
   ❑ The resident has a condition that may cause pain; history of pain
   ❑ Psychotropic side effects; other drug side effects
   ❑ Acute delirium and or confused state

2. **Pattern of above behavior/incidence:**

   Usual time of day (if any): _____

   Under what circumstances: _____

3. **Impaired communication:**

   ❑ Inability to speak or make needs known readily
   ❑ Inability to hear adequately
   ❑ Other: _____

4. **The following interventions have been attempted at this time, prior to restraint use:**

   ❑ Pain management
   ❑ Check for medication interaction(s)
   ❑ Check for underlying medical change/or subtle change in condition
   ❑ Toileting plan
   ❑ Ambulating regularly (place on ambulation program)

FIGURE B.2

Restraint needs assessment (cont.)

❏ Offer snacks, food

❏ Provide focused activity to divert resident (books, music, puzzles, etc.)

❏ Allow for naps

❏ Use tab monitors and other alarms

❏ Use fall mats or other (please list): _____

❏ Consult with rehab department for further direction (see PT eval)

5. **The following restraint** _____ **is determined for an initial trial period from** _____ **to** _____.

6. **The restraint elimination/reduction form will be used subsequently on a monthly basis.**

7. **Team signatures/titles/dates:**

    _____   _____   _____

    _____   _____   _____

FIGURE B.3

Incident/accident form

Name: _____
Room/Unit #: _____
Date: _____
Time: _____
Place: _____

Resident accident only
Indicate details of event:
❑ Found on floor ❑ Observed fall
❑ From bed ❑ From chair/wheelchair
Bed: ❑ High/regular ❑ Low
Side rails: ❑ Both up ❑ Both down ❑ 1 up
Call light used: ❑ Y ❑ N
Ambulatory: ❑ Y ❑ N
Significant medications:

_____
_____

Resident condition at time of discovery:
❑ Alert ❑ Confused ❑ Disoriented
❑ Combative ❑ Unconscious ❑ Visibly injured
Other: _____
Describe incident/discovery/history:

_____
_____
_____
_____

Describe disposition:

_____

Resolution:
❑ Remain in facility ❑ To ER for evaluation
❑ Admitted to hospital

Report to physician:
Physician name: _____
Date: _____ Time: _____
❑ Spoke to MD
❑ Left message with service

Report to family member:
Family member name: _____
Date: _____ Time: _____
❑ Spoke with family ❑ Left message to call

Notes:

_____
_____
_____
_____

Indicate site of injury:

Employee accident only: SS # _____-_____-_____   Position: _____ Dept: _____
Phone #: _____
Supervisor signature: _____
❑ Remained at work ❑ Sent home ❑ Sent for medical evaluation

I, _____ , refuse/accept medical treatment at this time:
        (employee name)

_____   _____
Signature/title   Date

Signature of person completing report	_____ Date _____ Time _____
Director of nursing	_____ Date _____
Medical director	_____ Date _____

FIGURE B.4

Pain management assessment form

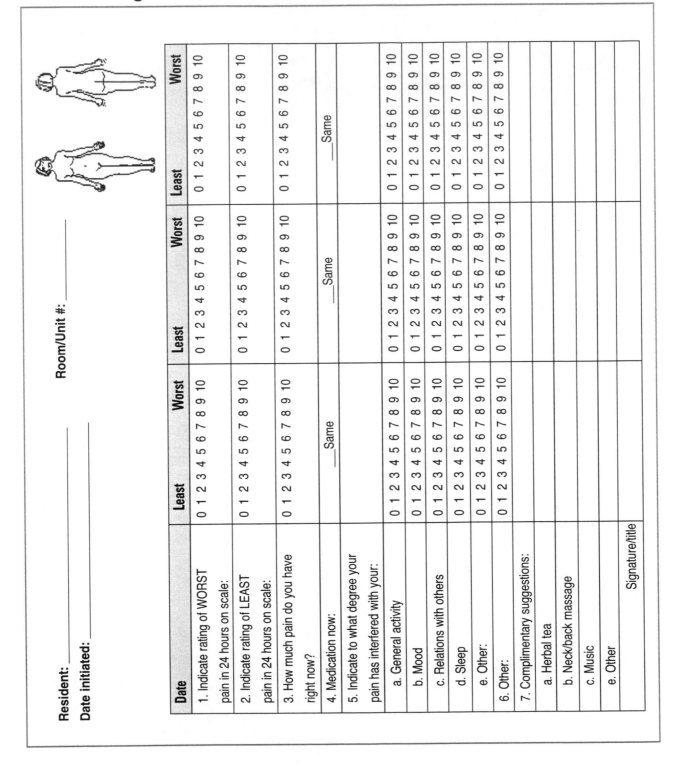

Resident: _____

Date initiated: _____

Room/Unit #: _____

Date	Least	Worst	Least	Worst	Least	Worst
1. Indicate rating of WORST pain in 24 hours on scale:	0 1 2 3 4 5 6 7 8 9 10		0 1 2 3 4 5 6 7 8 9 10		0 1 2 3 4 5 6 7 8 9 10	
2. Indicate rating of LEAST pain in 24 hours on scale:	0 1 2 3 4 5 6 7 8 9 10		0 1 2 3 4 5 6 7 8 9 10		0 1 2 3 4 5 6 7 8 9 10	
3. How much pain do you have right now?	0 1 2 3 4 5 6 7 8 9 10		0 1 2 3 4 5 6 7 8 9 10		0 1 2 3 4 5 6 7 8 9 10	
4. Medication now:	____ Same		____ Same		____ Same	
5. Indicate to what degree your pain has interfered with your:						
a. General activity	0 1 2 3 4 5 6 7 8 9 10		0 1 2 3 4 5 6 7 8 9 10		0 1 2 3 4 5 6 7 8 9 10	
b. Mood	0 1 2 3 4 5 6 7 8 9 10		0 1 2 3 4 5 6 7 8 9 10		0 1 2 3 4 5 6 7 8 9 10	
c. Relations with others	0 1 2 3 4 5 6 7 8 9 10		0 1 2 3 4 5 6 7 8 9 10		0 1 2 3 4 5 6 7 8 9 10	
d. Sleep	0 1 2 3 4 5 6 7 8 9 10		0 1 2 3 4 5 6 7 8 9 10		0 1 2 3 4 5 6 7 8 9 10	
e. Other:	0 1 2 3 4 5 6 7 8 9 10		0 1 2 3 4 5 6 7 8 9 10		0 1 2 3 4 5 6 7 8 9 10	
6. Other:	0 1 2 3 4 5 6 7 8 9 10		0 1 2 3 4 5 6 7 8 9 10		0 1 2 3 4 5 6 7 8 9 10	
7. Complimentary suggestions:						
a. Herbal tea						
b. Neck/back massage						
c. Music						
e. Other						
Signature/title						

FIGURE B.5

Assessment for bowel and bladder management

Resident Name _____

Room _____

DATE	DAY 1	DAY 2	DAY 3	DAY 4	DAY 5	DAY 6	DAY 7
7 AM							
8 AM							
9 AM							
10 AM							
11 AM							
12 PM							
1 PM							
2 PM							
3 PM							
4 PM							
5 PM							
6 PM							
7 PM							
8 PM							
9 PM							
10 PM							
11 PM							
12 AM							
1 AM							
2 AM							
3 AM							
4 AM							
5 AM							
6 AM							

Codes: **D** = DRY   **IBM** = INCONTINENT BM   **IU** = INCONTINENT URINE

TBM = TOILET BM   **TU** = TOILET URINE

FIGURE B.6

Pressure ulcer prevention measures

1. Systematically inspect skin daily. Pay particular attention to bony prominences. Document your findings. If skin is clear and intact, document the daily skin inspection by initialing a flow sheet.

2. Cleanse the skin with mild soap and water or a facility-approved product after each incontinence episode and at routine intervals. Avoid very hot water. Use a pH balanced product.

    *   Initiate an incontinence management or retraining program.
    *   Consider absorbent briefs or pads; use a good product that wicks moisture away from skin.
    *   Use an external catheter if necessary.
    *   Use an indwelling catheter only as a last resort.

3. Use moisturizers regularly to keep skin supple. Apply moisturizers after bathing to trap water in the upper layers of the skin, thus reducing dryness and itching. When choosing a moisturizer, look for products containing petrolatum, mineral oil, lanolin, ceramides, dimethicone, or glycerin. Avoid products containing alcohol, which is drying and irritating. Minimize environmental factors leading to drying. Many excellent barrier and protectant products are available to maintain skin integrity. Individualize the plan of care to the resident's needs. Products to consider are zinc oxide preparations, petrolatum- and silicone-based ointments and creams, liquid-forming products, adhesive dressings, fluid managers, skin cleansers, and moisturizers.

4. *Avoid massage over bony prominences and reddened areas.* This is an old treatment that is no longer recommended because it increases tissue destruction.

5. Apply barrier products to reduce skin exposure due to incontinence, perspiration, or wound drainage. Avoid powder or cornstarch, which can be irritating.

6. Avoid friction and shearing by using proper positioning, transferring, and turning techniques.

FIGURE B.6

Pressure ulcer prevention measures (cont.)

- **Friction** is rubbing the skin against a sheet or other surface.

- **Shearing** is moving the resident so the skin is stretched between the bone inside and the sheet (or other surface) outside, causing skin damage. The bone moves in one direction, whereas the skin stays stationary or moves in the opposite direction.

7. Provide adequate intake of fluid, protein, and calories. Monitor *and evaluate* intake and output for adequacy.

8. Improve the resident's mobility status if appropriate and as indicated.

9. Reposition residents every two hours or more often if indicated. Some residents may require positioning every 60–90 minutes.

10. Use props and positioning devices to keep bony prominences from direct contact with one another. If residents are positioned in bed with knees, ankles, and other bony areas touching each other, place bath blanket, pillow, or other positioning device between legs.

11. Keep heels elevated off the bed or hanging over the end of the mattress in bedfast residents. *Note:* Use of heel protectors reduces friction and shearing but does not relieve pressure. Avoid donut-type devices.

12. Avoid positioning directly on the trochanter. Use the semisupine and semiprone positions whenever possible. These are comfortable positions that relieve pressure on all major bony prominences.

13. Use lifting devices to move residents in bed whenever possible.

14. Maintain the head of the bed at the lowest degree of elevation possible (consistent with the resident's medical condition, physician orders, need for tube feeding, and other restrictions). Avoid elevations greater than 45 degrees as much as possible. Elevating the head of the

FIGURE B.6

Pressure ulcer prevention measures (cont.)

bed increases pressure on the sacrum, coccyx, and buttocks. If the head of the bed must be elevated for any reason, encourage or assist the resident to reposition frequently. Avoid prolonged periods of elevation.

15. Apply pressure-reducing mattresses and pads to bed and chair. The most common pressure-relieving devices are made of foam. Previously, sheepskin was thought to relieve pressure. Studies have shown that sheepskin prevents friction and shearing but does not relieve pressure.

16. Keep the bed-crumb and wrinkle-free.

17. Reposition chair-bound residents at least hourly. Teach residents to shift their weight every 15 minutes.

18. Provide education to other healthcare providers, residents, and family or caregivers about the prevention of pressure ulcers.

19. Provide adequate calories and protein to meet the resident's needs. Increase fluid intake. Provide supplements and snacks as ordered. Consider a dietician evaluation. Follow his or her recommendations. Monitor intake and output and meal and supplement intake when indicated.

20. Involve the resident in restorative nursing programs to maintain or improve his or her mobility and activity.

21. Monitor and document all interventions and outcomes.

22. Apply the principles of standard precautions if contact with blood, body fluids, secretions, excretions, mucous membranes, or nonintact skin is likely.

FIGURE B.6

Pressure ulcer prevention measures (cont.)

23. Institute an aggressive contracture prevention program. Involve other professionals (physical, occupational therapy and restorative nursing) as appropriate.

24. Weigh the resident. Monitor for significant weight loss (5% in 30 days; 10% in six months).

25. Monitor lab values for nutritional deficit:

    Hemoglobin <12mg/dl   Total lymphocyte count <1800 mm3

    Serum Albumin <3.5 mg/dl   Total Protein <6.0 mg/dl

26. Assess the need for vitamin/mineral supplements, such as multivitamin with minerals, vitamin C, and zinc, or as recommended by dietitian.

27. Educate staff! Most resident care is provided by nursing assistants. Make sure they understand aging changes to the skin, principles of "geriatric-friendly" skin care, safe transfer and repositioning techniques, methods of preventing and reducing friction and shearing, correct use of protective supplies (e.g., Geri gloves and sleeves, extremity stockinette, long sleeves, etc.) and equipment (e.g., padded side rails, wheelchairs arms, seats in good repair, etc.), how to report skin conditions to a nurse, signs and symptoms of infection, and expected wound appearance during the healing process.

FIGURE B.7

Fall assessment tool

Risk factor	Value	Assessment date	Score	Assessment date	Score	Assessment date	Score	Assessment date	Score
Alert, oriented, cooperative	0								
Uncooperative	2								
Confused, disoriented	4								
Unpredictable behavior	6								
Ambulatory independently (includes independent transfer and wheelchair propulsion)	0								
Siderails up in bed and/or transfers with assistance	2								
Ambulates with assistance or an assistive device	4								
Not ambulatory, immobile	6								
Previous history of falls	13								
Age under 51	0								
Age 51–60	2								
Age 61–70	4								
Over age 71 or mentally retarded	6								
No chemical restraint	0								
Receives prn medication that has the potential to decrease level of consciousness, or cause weakness	4								
Receives chemical restraint, sedative, or narcotic analgesic	6								
Total score									
Signature of assessor									

Total score 0–12 = low risk
Total score 13 or above = high risk

Note: The information listed here is for educational purposes only. Always follow your facility policies and procedures, physician orders, and state laws.